Dedication

This book is dedicated to my husband, Bill; our adult children, Zandy and Libby; our children-in-law, Heidi and Lee; our grandchildren, Hayden and Liam Garrard and Henry and Helen Glascoe; and our energetic canine companion, Sophie.

FIFTH EDITION

Health Sciences Literature Review Made Easy

THE MATRIX METHOD

JUDITH GARRARD, PHD

Professor Emeritus
School of Public Health
University of Minnesota
Minneapolis, Minnesota

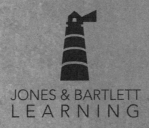

JONES & BARTLETT
L E A R N I N G

World Headquarters
Jones & Bartlett Learning
5 Wall Street
Burlington, MA 01803
978-443-5000
info@jblearning.com
www.jblearning.com

Jones & Bartlett Learning books and products are available through most bookstores and online booksellers. To contact Jones & Bartlett Learning directly, call 800-832-0034, fax 978-443-8000, or visit our website, www.jblearning.com.

Substantial discounts on bulk quantities of Jones & Bartlett Learning publications are available to corporations, professional associations, and other qualified organizations. For details and specific discount information, contact the special sales department at Jones & Bartlett Learning via the above contact information or send an email to specialsales@jblearning.com.

Production Credits

VP, Executive Publisher: David D. Cella
Executive Editor: Amanda Martin
Associate Acquisitions Editor: Rebecca Stephenson
Associate Editor: Danielle Bessette
Production Editor: Vanessa Richards
Senior Marketing Manager: Jennifer Scherzay
Product Fulfillment Manager: Wendy Kilborn

Composition: S4Carlisle Publishing Services
Cover Design: Kristin E. Parker
Rights & Media Specialist: Jamey O'Quinn
Media Development Editor: Troy Liston
Cover Image: © Attitude/Shutterstock
Printing and Binding: Edwards Brothers Malloy
Cover Printing: Edwards Brothers Malloy

To order this product, use ISBN: 9781284115192

Library of Congress Cataloging-in-Publication Data
Names: Garrard, Judith, author.
Title: Health sciences literature review made easy : the matrix method /
    Judith Garrard.
Description: Fifth edition. | Burlington, Massachusetts : Jones & Bartlett
    Learning, [2017] | Includes bibliographical references and index.
Identifiers: LCCN 2016010950 | ISBN 9781284133950 (pbk.)
Subjects: | MESH: Review Literature as Topic | Medical Writing | Abstracting
    and Indexing as Topic | Information Storage and Retrieval
Classification: LCC R118.6 | NLM WZ 345 | DDC 610.72--dc23 LC record available at
    http://lccn.loc.gov/2016010950

6048

Printed in the United States of America
20 19 18 17 16   10 9 8 7 6 5 4 3 2 1

Contents

Preface

Health Sciences Literature Review Made Easy: The Matrix Method, Fifth Edition has a number of additions and changes. Here is a summary:

- **Research Synthesis**: Chapter 1 has been expanded, with a more detailed discussion of the research synthesis field, especially the guidelines for reporting better studies and the guidelines for expert-led reviews. Also included are websites to help students stay up to date in future developments in the field of research synthesis.
- **Web-Based Tutorials**: In Chapter 2 under "Citations, References, Bibliographies," I provided instructions for accessing web-based tutorials on the use of APA and AMA styles of citation for almost any type of reference needed in writing a synthesis of the literature.
- **PRISMA Flowchart**: The use of the PRISMA Flowchart of Number of Documents from Initiation to Completion of Review has been emphasized in Chapter 1 and has become an important complement to the Matrix Method in Chapters 4 and 6.
- **Exercises for Student Review**: A new section, "What You Should Know or Be Able to Do by the End of This Chapter," has been added at the end of Chapters 1 through 6. These could serve as faculty-assigned exercises or be used by students either individually or in study groups.
- **Master Folder**: I modified the label, Lit Review Master Folder, which I now call the Master Folder. I also clarified how to better label the Master Folders if the reader has more than one. This change was made throughout the book.
- **Organizing the Folders**: In Chapters 3 through 6, I have a section on how to organize each folder: Paper Trail Folder, Documents Folder, Review

Matrix Folder, and Synthesis Folder, all stored in the Master Folder. This should help readers better organize their own files.

- **Writing the Synthesis**: I expanded Chapter 6 on how to write a synthesis of the literature. There is also a new section on papers published in nursing journals of a research synthesis in Chapter 6 based on publications in the peer-reviewed literature that used both the Matrix Method and an adaptation of the PRISMA Flowchart of documents from initiation to completion of review. These three publications are excellent examples that can be used by students to guide their own preparation of a synthesis.

- **More Hints and Examples**: Throughout Chapters 1 through 6, I added more hints to help students with practical advice. Each hint is in a box to help easily identify them.

- **Caroline's Quest**: These descriptions about the process of using the Matrix Method in Chapters 1 through 6 have been brought up to date by incorporating the additions and changes in the fifth edition.

The *Fourth Edition* included the creation of two new sections and some chapters were expanded, all of which are included in the *Fifth Edition*. The following were the new sections:

- **Methodological Review of the Literature**: This section in Chapter 2 has been completely rewritten for the *Fourth Edition*. A new visual, the Methods Map, was used for the first time in the book. The description of the Methods Map follows a logical progression in the analysis of a study: from statement of the initial question, through generation of a random sample, layout of the methodological design, final interpretation of statistical results, and application of answers to the initial research question.

- **Appendix C, Data Visualization: A Digital Exploration**: Not only is this a new topic for this book but how it is offered is also new. Jones & Bartlett Learning made it possible to offer this exciting topic in a digital environment. How else would you see the range of possibilities for data visualization if not in the environment for which it was intended? I urge you to go there now to begin this exploration. An Online Access Code unique to each copy of the book is required to access the Appendix and you can return repeatedly to Appendix C by using that code.

The *Third Edition* included the following revisions:

- **Electronic Basis**: The Matrix Method has been converted from a hard copy method (using three-ring notebooks and paper-based spreadsheets) to an entirely electronic basis (including computer folders and subfolders).

An appendix serves as a guide for setting up such files, and information is interwoven throughout all the chapters that describe this move to an electronic basis.

- **National Library of Medicine**: This edition describes the rapidly changing innovations in the National Library of Medicine infrastructure and the impact of these changes on how to review the literature in the health sciences.
- **Changes in the Field**: Different terms have been introduced to describe a review of the literature These terms and how they compare to the kind of literature review described in this book are presented.

The purpose, scope, and emphasis of the text have not changed from the initial publication of this book to this *Fifth Edition*. They remain as follows:

- **Purpose**: The purpose of this book is to describe a practical and useful method for reviewing the literature, especially the scientific literature in the health sciences. The audience continues to be graduate or professional students who need a practical, step-by-step set of instructions for how to conduct a review of the literature. That is its fundamental goal.
- **Scope**: The scope of this text spans from beginning students to health professionals in the workplace The methods for conducting a review of the literature apply to all major health professions, including public health, nursing, dentistry, medicine, pharmacy, veterinary medicine, and the allied health sciences.
- **Emphasis**: The emphasis in this text is on practical applications. My goal was and continues to be a method for actually conducting a review of the literature and preparing a narrative synthesis.

Acknowledgments

With each new edition of this text, I have had the pleasure of working with colleagues from my past and new experts, all of whom have been exciting to work with. For the *Fifth Edition*, I called on an old friend, Del Reed, PhD, who is a reference librarian in the University of Minnesota's Biomedical Library. He answered a variety of questions as I wrote this current edition. In writing the expanded section on research synthesis in Chapter 1, I had the help of colleagues from my past: Sue Duval, PhD, Associate Professor, School of Medicine, whose expertise is in meta analysis, and Mary Butler, PhD, Assistant Professor and Associate Director of the Minnesota Evidence-Based Practice Center in the School of Public Health; both are at the University of Minnesota. Finally, through the efforts of Rebecca Stephenson at Jones & Bartlett Learning, three reviewers in nursing volunteered to let me interview them about how they used the book and what they needed for the new edition. Thank you to Rodney Hicks, Professor, College of Graduate Nursing, Western University of Health Sciences, Pomona, California, and Cynthia S. Jacelon, PhD, Professor and Director of the PhD Program, School of Nursing, University of Massachusetts, Amherst, Massachusetts. What these two professors are doing to teach the science of research synthesis to their nursing students, including the use of the Matrix Method, is inspiring! I also appreciate the willingness of Jacqueline M. McGrath, PhD, Associate Dean, University of Connecticut School of Nursing, Storrs, Connecticut, to be interviewed; unfortunately, my travel schedule did not make this possible.

As this edition has moved from my writing to eventually the hands of readers, I am especially grateful to my editor, Rebecca Stephenson, for her guidance and active involvement in producing this *Fifth Edition* and to the associate editor,

Danielle Bessette. The extensive copyediting and proofreading of this *Fifth Edition* has been made possible by the very professional team led by Vanessa Richards, Production Editor, her colleague, Jamey O'Quinn, Rights & Media Specialist, both at Jones & Bartlett Learning, and Manjusha Chandrasekaran, Project Manager for the copyediting, typesetting, and proofreading stages of the book at S4Carlisle Publishing Services.

In the *Fourth Edition*, I greatly benefited from the advice and guidance of the Digital Learning Group (DLG) in the School of Public Health, University of Minnesota as I developed Appendix C. In particular, my guide throughout the development of the electronic aspects of this edition has been Bernadette Gloeb, MLS, an Instructional Designer in the DLG. She has provided inspiration, skills in transitioning from ideas to practical designs, and especially enthusiasm for the digital aspects of our work together.

The *Third Edition* reflected the many changes in tools researchers use to develop a literature review and how those tools are typically used. Some of the most dramatic changes have been in the resources available in university-based biomedical libraries.

In preparing the *Third Edition*, I had the good fortune to work with three dynamic biomedical librarians at the University of Minnesota Health Sciences Libraries in the preparation of these materials, and I want to gratefully acknowledge them: Chad Fennel, Lisa McGuire, and Del Reed. During the months that we met, they taught me a lot about the present and future resources in today's health sciences libraries, and I want to urge the readers of this text to seek out their own equivalent of this dynamic group of librarians at their own libraries.

The *Second Edition* and *Third Edition* would not have been possible without a *First Edition*, and I am continually grateful for the help from another librarian, Julie Kelly, at the University of Minnesota's Magrath Library. The improvements and additions to the *Second Edition* reflect input from all of these people; the errors are mine alone.

I also want to acknowledge the continued support and encouragement of my husband, Bill Garrard, in this endeavor, as well as that of our children, their spouses, and our grandchildren (and our canine companions).

My editors and their colleagues at Jones & Bartlett Learning have been patient and encouraging throughout the process of completion of the *Fifth Edition*, just as they were for the previous editions.

About the Author

Judith Garrard, PhD, retired from the University of Minnesota in January 2015, and is now a professor emeritus. During her 44 years as a faculty member in the health sciences and a professor in the School of Public Health at the University of Minnesota, she was a research psychologist with postgraduate training in epidemiology.

Her teaching and research activities were on a multidisciplinary basis throughout her career. For more than 35 years she taught graduate courses in research and program evaluation methods to students in public health, nursing, medicine, dentistry, veterinary medicine, and pharmacy, as well as those in education, psychology, and social work.

Dr. Garrard's research specialty was pharmacoepidemiology and patient outcomes, with a focus on prescription drug use by elderly people in the community, nursing homes, and assisted living facilities. She has authored or coauthored over 100 papers and reports, including peer-reviewed research papers on psychotropic drug use by elderly people. Over the past 10 years, she was one of four co-investigators in an NINDS-funded Research Center, based in the School of Pharmacy. Her specialty was epidemiological research on the use of antiepileptic drug use by nursing home residents, in collaboration with colleagues in pharmacy, neurology, and biostatistics. She has also been principal investigator or collaborator on numerous multidisciplinary research projects supported by NIH grants from the National Institute on Aging, National Institute for Neurological Diseases and Stroke, National Institute on Nursing, Agency for Health Care Policy Research, Health Care Financing Administration, Veterans Administration, and other granting agencies.

In 1990, Dr. Garrard received the Leonard M. Schuman Excellence in Teaching Award, and in 1991 a Career Research Award in social and behavioral geriatrics from the National Institute on Aging, NIH. In 1999, her book, *Health Sciences Literature Review Made Easy: The Matrix Method*, was published by Aspen Publications, Inc. The *Second, Third*, and *Fourth Editions* were published by Jones & Bartlett Learning in 2007, 2010, 2013, respectively; this is the *Fifth Edition*. She can be reached by email at the following address: jgarrard@umn.edu.

Fundamentals of a Literature Review

Part I is an introduction to basic terminology, the field of research synthesis, and tutorials to get you started. It consists of two chapters that cover the basic terms and content you will need in order to understand how to use The Matrix Method.

Chapter 1, *Introduction*, defines what is meant by a review of the literature, describes the broader field of research synthesis, and discusses two internationally developed guidelines, one for designing better studies and the second for expert led reviews. A new feature, the PRISMA Flowchart, is introduced in the *Fifth Edition* as a complement to The Matrix Method that emphasizes better clarification of the literature reviewed.

Chapter 2, *Basic Concepts*, focuses on some of the fundamental information you will need to conduct your own review of the literature. Specifically, basic concepts are defined, the anatomy of a typical health sciences journal article is described, and a tutorial is presented on how to conduct a methodological review, which is one part of a review of the literature.

Caroline's Quest is an ongoing section in each chapter. Its purpose is to demonstrate the process of understanding and applying the content of each chapter.

What You Should Know or Be Able to Do by the End of This Chapter, another new feature of the *Fifth Edition,* is included at the end of both chapters. Test yourself with these questions to determine whether you really did know what was covered.

CHAPTER 1

Introduction

The Matrix Method is a versatile way to review the literature. The background and philosophy of a literature review and an introduction to the Matrix Method are described in the following sections in this chapter:

- Review of the Literature
- Well Beyond Index Cards
- To Own the Literature
- Research Synthesis: Historical Perspective
- Guidelines for Designing and Reporting Better Studies
- Guidelines for Expert-Led Reviews
- PRISMA, PROSPERO and a Journal
- IOM Standards for Systematic Reviews: Finding What Works in Health Care
- Scoping Reviews: Finding the Gaps in Existing Literature
- Future Guidelines and Revisions in the Health Sciences Literature
- Difference Between Systematic Reviews, Scoping Reviews, and Reviews of the Literature
- The Matrix Method: Definition and Overview
- Review Matrix: A Versatile Tool
- Overview of Chapters and Appendices
- References to Websites
- Caroline's Quest: Understanding the Process
- What You Should Know or Be Able to Do by the End of This Chapter

REVIEW OF THE LITERATURE

The purpose of this book is to describe the Matrix Method and the Matrix Indexing System. The Matrix Method is a strategy for reviewing the literature, especially the scientific literature. A review of the literature consists of reading, analyzing, and writing a synthesis of scholarly materials about a specific topic. When the review is of scientific literature, the focus is on the hypotheses, the scientific methods, the strengths and weaknesses of the study, the results, and the authors' interpretations and conclusions. A review of the scientific literature is fundamental to understanding the accumulated knowledge about the topic being reviewed. The Matrix Indexing System helps the user create and maintain an electronic reprint file.

The term *scientific literature* refers to theoretical and research publications in scientific journals, reference books, textbooks, government reports, policy statements, and other materials about the theory, practice, and results of scientific inquiry. These materials and publications are produced by individuals or groups in universities, foundations, government research laboratories, and other non-profit or for-profit organizations. Throughout this text, the term *source document* will be used to refer to any of these sources, such as a journal article, a chapter in a book, or a research report. Currently, the most common type of publication used in a review of up-to-date scientific literature is a research paper in a scientific journal, such as the *Journal of the American Medical Association* (*JAMA*) or the *American Journal of Epidemiology*.

Reviews of the literature are the foundation for theses and dissertations, grant proposals, research papers, summary articles, books, policy and regulatory statements, evidence-based healthcare statements for health professionals, and consumer materials. Given the vast number of scientific publications produced over the past several decades, information retrieval and analysis in the form of a critical review of the literature have become more crucial than ever.

Over the past 20–30 years, the following terms have been used interchangeably: literature review, integrative review, systematic review, and meta-analysis. All share the same basic elements: (1) stating the purpose of the review; (2) screening and selecting scientific papers that meet specified criteria; (3) carefully reviewing the papers for excellence of scientific methods, statistical procedures, and validity and reliability of data collection; (4) summarizing findings across the studies; and (5) drawing conclusions based on the scientific evidence.

In this book, a *literature review* is defined as an analysis of scientific materials about a specific topic that requires the reviewer to carefully read each of the studies to evaluate the study purpose, determine the appropriateness and quality of the scientific methods, examine the analysis of the questions and answers posed by the authors, summarize the findings across the studies, and write an objective synthesis of the findings.

In describing an integrative review, authors emphasize the review of past research in which the goal of the review is to base conclusions on many different studies.[1] Although *integrative review* (or *integrative literature review*) is a term that tended to be found in the nursing literature, it now has broader appeal. An integrative review aims to synthesize the literature from the past with the current literature and to draw logical and useful conclusions.

The term *systematic review* appears more frequently in publications about evidence-based medicine. The term has been defined as an overview of scientific evidence in the medical literature that emphasizes treatment, causation, diagnosis, and prognosis.[2] According to this definition, systematic reviews are prepared specifically for clinicians and provide the basis for the practice of evidence-based medicine. Other clinical fields have adopted the strategy of basing their clinical practices and decision-making processes on the evidence in the scientific literature.

Beginning in the early 2000s, the term *systematic review* was redefined in the growing field of research synthesis. Currently, *systematic review or meta-analysis* has a specific meaning tied to the use of guidelines for expert-led reviews issued by the Cochrane Collaboration or in the 2009 PRISMA Statement[3] or the 2011 IOM Standards for Systematic Reviews.[4]

A *meta-analysis* is a departure from the other three types of reviews because this kind of literature summary requires precise quantitative methods to summarize the results. The same standards of rigor in identifying the purpose of the review, careful selection of papers, and evaluation of methods are essential to this type of review.

In general, think about the first three types of reviews as being similar, with the names being used in specific fields or disciplines to basically refer to a very rigorous literature review. The meta-analysis is described more fully later in this text.

WELL BEYOND INDEX CARDS

Prior to the widespread availability of computers, many students conducted their first review of the literature in high school or in college when they learned how to do library research. Usually, they concentrated on where to gather information and how to use the library. With the advent of computers, students now learn about electronic information retrieval at the primary school level.

Using computers to retrieve information is not the only new development, however. The sheer amount of information to be examined and critiqued has increased exponentially over the past 50 years. The first decade of the 21st century alone witnessed tremendous advancements in scientific knowledge, a dramatic increase in the number of scientific journals, and a bewildering array of new forms of communication. Books and scientific journals are no longer the only venues for scholarly literature. Information is available on the Internet, in national and international meetings of professional societies, and in correspondence by email, on blogs, and through social networking software such as Twitter, Facebook, and wikis. The issue of how, where, when, and whether or not to obtain information from these sources constitutes a present-day dilemma for anyone who reviews the scientific literature. The art of conducting such a review is an entirely separate matter.

In the past, American students were advised to use index cards to record the most salient points of the material being reviewed. Now students keep notes on a computer or on other electronic devices. Despite such technological advances, how to avoid getting lost in the details between generating a computer list of research articles, accumulating electronic notes, and writing the final synthesis is still something of a mystery to many people.

One way to master this process is to realize that a review of any body of literature actually consists of four fundamental tasks, after the subject of the review has been decided:

1. Make decisions about which documents to review.
2. Read and understand what the authors describe in those documents.
3. Evaluate the ideas, research methods, and results of each publication.
4. Write a synthesis that includes both the content and a critical analysis of these materials.

Given the complexity of each one of these tasks, it is easy to become overwhelmed in the process. A strategy is needed to organize the books and papers selected in the search and retrieval process, structure the information in order to understand the progression of ideas by different authors across documents and over time, and use that structure to develop a critique and write a synthesis of the results of such a review. The Matrix Method provides such a strategy.

TO OWN THE LITERATURE

Something else can result from a thorough and comprehensive review of the literature that may be even more valuable than a written synthesis—ownership of the literature. To own the literature you must know it—know the major ideas, what has been researched, the names of the authors and their professional affiliations, who collaborated with whom, what databases they did (or did not) use, the methodological strengths and weaknesses of the studies, what has been studied ad infinitum, and especially what is missing.

To own the literature is to be so familiar with what has been written by previous researchers that you know clearly how this area of research has progressed over time and across ideas. Without a thorough and comprehensive review of the literature, you are at the mercy of every critic and reviewer who is aware of what is known, how it evolved, and what has yet to be examined.

Unfortunately, such ownership cannot be acquired easily; you have to complete the entire process of a literature review, from the initial search to the final written synthesis, before you can take possession of the literature on a subject. Ownership is rarely mentioned when people describe the literature in a paper or presentation, but it exists; experienced reviewers achieve such ownership whether or not they realize it.

When you own the literature, you are in a better position to know what is missing in a stream of research. You can defend your ideas and anticipate what other scientists and researchers will say or do. Ownership is the mastery of how a specific body of knowledge evolved, what it currently comprises, and what has yet to be studied.

Acquiring ownership of the literature demands more than summarizing the studies or documents you reviewed. A summary merely describes. Your task is to read and analyze each document until you can picture what the authors did in a study or the logical process they went through in making a point. Then you must go back and critically analyze what was right and wrong each step of the way. To own the literature is to dissect each part of it and decide whether you agree with what the authors did or said. In other words, you must become engaged with the content, argue with the authors' logic, and conclude for yourself whether that paper or study made sense from a scientific or scholarly standpoint. You must understand how the field has evolved, including the progression of ideas over time and across different authors. To own the literature you must learn about the conceptual models that served as the foundation for the research, and you must deduce what hypotheses were really being tested, who initiated the ideas, and who did the first research study. The Matrix Method will help you acquire ownership of the literature, but it is only a guide. The most important component is your active involvement with the literature.

RESEARCH SYNTHESIS: HISTORICAL PERSPECTIVE

Overview

Before delving into the details of the Matrix Method, it might be useful to think about the historical context of a literature review. A literature review is part of the larger endeavor of research synthesis, which is the analysis, interpretation, and use of scientific inquiry. Although the term *research synthesis* can be applied to all kinds of knowledge, this discussion is limited to examples of how the synthesis of health sciences research literature has evolved. The practices and tools used today for reviewing the health sciences literature can be traced back to 1879 with the publication of *Index Medicus*, a medical bibliography that included a subject and author index to articles published in medical journals.[5] Today's most useful tools, however, are relatively recent innovations. A historical awareness of how the research literature has grown and when some of these tools were introduced will help put these developments into perspective.

Since the mid-1940s, the number of scientific publications has increased dramatically. What spurred this increase is complicated and best left to social and medical historians to explain, but certainly a major factor has been a concomitant rise in the amount of funding for research by the National Institutes of Health (NIH). These growth rates are shown in **Figure 1-1**. In this example, publications are those defined by the Science Citation Index as original substantive articles, editorial materials, letters, reports of meetings, correction notes, and reviews for the period from 1945 to 1996.[6,7] The NIH dollars are those allocated for research grants.[8]

Some critics suggest that there is no evidence of an increase in the rate of scientific publications over time, citing the following two reasons for this rationale: (1) the quantity of scientific publications has increased, but the quality has not,[9] and (2) the rate of publications per health scientist has remained the same, but the number of health scientists has increased.[10] Neither argument addresses the fact that scholars today must cope with an increase in the absolute number of journals and publications that must be considered when reviewing the literature.

In examining the growth rates in Figure 1-1, the increase in NIH grant dollars may not be as steep as indicated because the figures are actual dollars spent for each 5-year period, unadjusted for inflation. The real rate of growth may be flatter or dip more in some years than others, after inflation has been taken into account. For the sake of argument, however, consider the two rates of growth at their face value, and assume an upward trajectory for both.

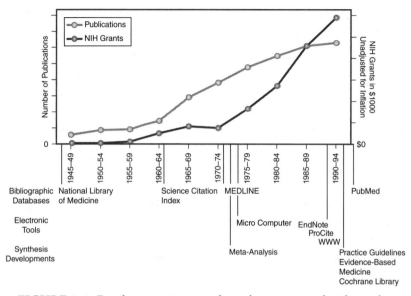

FIGURE 1-1 Developments in research synthesis compared with number of scientific publications and funding for research grants from the NIH

Data about publications are from Institute for Scientific Information. Science citation index 1945–1954: cumulative comparative statistical summary. In: *SCI Science Citation Index Ten Year Cumulation 1945–1954: Guide and Lists of Source Publications.* Vol 8. Philadelphia, PA: Institute for Scientific Information; 1988:18–19[6]; Institute for Scientific Information. Comparative statistical summary 1955–1996. In: *SCI Science Citation Index 1996 Annual Guide and Lists of Source Publications.* Vol 1. Philadelphia, PA: Institute for Scientific Information; 1997:57–63[7]; Institute for Scientific Information. Data about NIH research funds are from National Institutes of Health. *NIH Almanac 1997.* Washington, DC: National Institutes of Health; 1997. NIH Publication No. 97-5.[8]

What is important is the juxtaposition of the growth in the number of publications, the amount of research funding, and developments in resources for creating a synthesis of the research literature. Examples of these developments over the past 50 years can be assigned to three categories: (1) the establishment of bibliographic databases, (2) the availability of electronic tools for manipulating information, and (3) the emergence of synthesis applications.

Bibliographic Databases

Bibliographic databases include information in print and electronic forms. The first major development in this category for the health sciences was the creation of the National Library of Medicine (NLM) under the aegis of the Public Health Service of the Department of Health, Education, and Welfare. The NLM evolved from the Library of the Army Surgeon General's Office, which was established in 1836.[5] With major funding from Congress in 1942, the NLM gathered a national collection of scientific books, papers, and reports located in Washington, DC. Accessing this information electronically was difficult for scientists in other parts of the country; this was only partially solved in 1961 with the creation of the Science Citation Index and later its sister application, the Social Science Citation Index, by Eugene Garfield, PhD.[11] These indexes, owned and published by the Institute for Scientific Information, were acquired by Thomson Scientific in 1992.

In 1971, MEDLINE, an electronic database of the scientific literature in medical and other health-related journals and publications, was launched by the NLM and became one of the premier tools for health sciences researchers. Initially, access to MEDLINE was brokered by reference librarians, which made frequent or spontaneous use awkward in the daily life of most scientists. Such use could also be expensive, and a charge per reference had a chilling effect on financially strapped graduate students and unfunded assistant professors—the very users who most needed such access.

The rules for searching MEDLINE were also complicated. Reference librarians had to undergo specialized training to master the intricacies of the search, and not all research libraries had specialized personnel. Nonetheless, the availability of an electronic database that could be searched to locate specific studies was a major advantage for health scientists engaged in research synthesis.

Gradually, an infrastructure for an electronic bibliographic database became more refined, with standardized keywords and more easily understood rules for creating a search strategy. Although scientists intent on using the electronic version of MEDLINE were still bound to one of the research libraries, and bound even more tightly to the services of a knowledgeable librarian, this ability to access the research literature was a major advantage. The number of research publications had already begun an upswing by this point in time. This is reflected in the rate of growth shown in Figure 1-1 for the period after MEDLINE became available, although cause and effect have not been clearly established between the development and the rate.

The period since MEDLINE's inception has seen the creation of myriad other bibliographic databases, such as PsycINFO (Psychological Information database produced by the American Psychological Association), International Pharmaceutical Abstracts, and CINAHL (Cumulative Index to Nursing and Allied Health Literature). Two additional bibliographic databases were launched around the turn of the 21st century: PubMed in 1997 and PubMed Central in 2008.

PubMed, based in the NLM, provides worldwide access to MEDLINE on the Internet. Anyone—scientist or layperson—now has access to the MEDLINE database of over 18 million references just by signing onto its website. Not only is PubMed free, but the use of MEDLINE is no longer tied geographically to a library or restricted to the availability of a qualified librarian. All that is needed is a computer and access to the Internet.

PubMed Central, a part of the NIH, is a free digital archive of biomedical and life sciences literature. The goal of PubMed Central is to provide full-text papers, not just abstracts, of scientific research funded by the NIH. These two databases, PubMed and PubMed Central, are interrelated, and together they provide rapid access to research publications.

Electronic Tools

Only a few examples of developments in the second category, electronic tools, are described here, beginning with the microcomputer. Without a doubt, the introduction in the mid-1970s of a reasonably priced personal computer represents a seminal event in any historical description of the late 20th century. For reviewers of the literature, the availability of a personal computer vastly improved the quality of scholarly life. Word processing software, together with information in bibliographic databases, made the tasks of searching and abstracting the scientific literature far more efficient.

There continued to be other problems, however, one of which was the lack of a standardized format for citations and references to articles in scientific journals or books. If a health scientist had to switch from one formatting system, such as the APA system, to another (e.g., the AMA system), in the preparation of a paper or report, then he or she was forced to go back through the entire document and make the changes one by one. Although there is still no single, universal format, another kind of solution was developed. In the late 1980s, two reference management software packages were produced that automatically made changes from one formatting system to another, thus providing some relief for time-strapped researchers. Academicians created both software products—EndNote in 1988, and ProCite in 1989.

RefWorks, introduced in 2002, is a web-based product that is generally available to faculty and students through an institutional subscription at university and college libraries. Not only do these software packages satisfy their original intent of allowing the user to switch from one reference formatting system to another, but they now have additional features such as the creation of a reference library on the user's own computer or web-based document, a search and sort capability, the seamless download of a reference and its abstract from electronic bibliographic databases to desktop computers, and the flexibility of user-defined information for each reference.

The impact of reference management software packages does not equal that of the personal computer in a list of important developments in the history of research synthesis or information management. Nevertheless, these software products are good, solid tools for everyday use and are like a set of well-honed kitchen utensils compared with the discovery of fire—the latter is necessary, but after that is available, the former makes the job easier.

Like the personal computer, another advance comparable to the discovery of fire was the establishment of the World Wide Web in 1989. With the Web, individual researchers have free and unlimited worldwide access to fellow researchers and also to multiple banks of information such as the electronic bibliographic databases and other scientific forums that have rapidly proliferated. The use of these electronic tools in combination with bibliographic databases, together with an increase in the absolute number of scientific publications and NIH grant dollars, contributed to developments in the third category of development: synthesis applications.

Synthesis Applications

It is easy to imagine that if the same rate of growth in scientific publications had been seen in the financial market, investors would have been ecstatic. There was more research, better science, and an exponential growth in new information, but the scientific community pondered how to make use of it. How could this growing reservoir of scientific knowledge be managed and used for the betterment of humankind or, at least, for individual patients? Three developments in the late 1990s illustrate a response to these issues: practice guidelines, evidence-based medicine, and the Cochrane reviews of clinical trials. These developments are shown at the far right of the timeline in Figure 1-1. Prior to their appearance, however, a new methodological technique, meta-analysis, was proposed in the mid-1970s, just before personal computers and the Web became available.

Meta-Analysis

Gene Glass, a professor of education, was one of the first to outline a way of statistically summarizing the results of multiple studies on the same topic. His initial paper was published in 1976.[12] Health scientists quickly saw the advantage of this technique and began to apply it to biomedical research studies. The use of this and other techniques contributed to the development of the following prime examples of synthesis applications in the 1990s:

- Clinical practice guidelines generated largely by the Americans
- Evidence-based medicine created by the Canadians
- Reviews by the worldwide Cochrane Collaboration led by the British

All of these resulted from national and international collaborations, made possible by local, national, and international funding. These developments depend on the resources of bibliographic databases, electronic tools, and an intense commitment to making use of available research findings to improve the health care of individuals and the public.

Clinical Practice Guidelines

Practice guidelines were developed with the intention of providing practitioners, such as physicians, nurses, and allied health professionals, with sound strategies based on the scientific literature for delivering the best possible health care. A formal definition of a clinical practice guideline was provided by the Institute of Medicine (IOM) in 1992.[13]

In 1993, the first practice guideline was commissioned and funded by the Agency for Health Care Policy and Research (AHCPR), a federal granting agency created by Congress in 1989. Over the following 5 years, AHCPR commissioned practice guidelines on 19 topics that were published between 1992 and 1998. Examples of topics include acute pain management, depression in primary care, HIV infection, otitis media with effusion in children, and poststroke rehabilitation.

In conjunction with the American Association of Health Plans and the American Medical Association, AHCPR developed the National Guideline Clearinghouse website, http://www.guideline.gov, dedicated to enhancing access to the guidelines in 1998. The current successor of AHCPR is the AHRQ (Agency for Healthcare Research and Quality), which has redefined its role as the facilitator to other organizations, such as specialty societies, managed care organizations or local groups of clinicians, in their development of future practice guidelines.

Evidence-Based Medicine

The basic concepts of evidence-based medicine were conceived by a group of academicians at McMaster University in Hamilton, Ontario, led by Professor G. H. Guyatt. The medical school at McMaster has long been known for its innovativeness in medical education, and these clinician–scholars expanded their audience from a classroom of medical students in southern Canada to healthcare providers throughout the world.

Guyatt and his colleagues recognized the need for members of the medical community to improve their ability to evaluate and use the scientific literature.[11]

An ongoing series of Users Guides to the Medical Literature, published in *JAMA*, has provided a set of tutorials for clinicians on such diverse topics as how to use articles about diagnosis, prognosis, grading healthcare recommendations, and applicability of clinical trial results. A list of such articles from 1993 to 2000 is provided in the references section at the end of this chapter[14-46] and also by year of publication in Appendix A. The concepts of evidence-based medicine have been adopted by clinicians in other disciplines, including nursing, dentistry, and pharmacy. A term with broader application has begun to emerge— *evidence-based practice*. The relationship between evidence-based practice and clinical practice guidelines has not been fully examined, although logically they are closely linked. Clearly, what they have in common is a foundation of scientific literature that has been carefully reviewed and systematically abstracted. At its simplest, evidence-based practice is what a practitioner such as a physician or nurse–clinician does one-on-one with a patient, whereas practice guidelines provide guidance for best clinical practice.

The Cochrane Collaboration

In 1992, a nonprofit organization, the Cochrane Centre, was created in Oxford, England, in response to concerns expressed 20 years earlier by Archie Cochrane, a British epidemiologist.[58] An outgrowth of the Centre was the establishment in 1993 of the Cochrane Collaboration, an international, voluntary, collaborative effort to provide systematic and critical reviews of RCTs of health care.[59] Participants in the collaboration are organized through collaborative review groups that include researchers, healthcare professionals, and consumers throughout the world, including experts in the United States and Canada.

The ongoing mission of the Cochrane Collaboration is to prepare, maintain, and promote the accessibility of systematic reviews of the effects of healthcare interventions. Current information about the Cochrane Collaboration in the United States can be found at http://us.cochrane.org.

Results of reviews of empirical studies by the Cochrane Collaboration are maintained in the Cochrane Library, in which communication is rapid and easily accessible via the Internet. Lay audiences can readily obtain the reviews themselves. Thus, the Cochrane Library has an important role to play in the democratization of healthcare information. The availability of the Cochrane Library dates back to the mid-1990s. The further development and impact of this resource for health professionals, policy makers, and consumers bear close scrutiny in the future.

This brief history of the emergence of the field of research synthesis in the health sciences has focused exclusively on developments in English language systems, and largely in North America, with some mention of the role of the British. Linguistic and geographic boundaries of science are disappearing daily, however, and the full scope of developments and use of research synthesis cannot be confined to a single language or these few countries. Globalization exists in the scientific arena, including the private sector.

Initially, the Cochrane Collaboration limited their focus to a synthesis of studies that used randomized clinical/controlled trials (RCTs). But a field of scientific inquiry needed to have matured to have a sufficient number of RCT papers available to make possible such a review. Although many fields had not reached that point, other scholars, scientists, practitioners, and the public still needed expert reviews of the current literature. By 2004, the Cochrane Collaboration broadened its methodological criteria to include reviews of scientific papers using non-RCTs or observational methods.

In the future, the history of research synthesis will need a broader cultural and linguistic perspective to provide a complete understanding of the impact of this discipline on the health of people. The role of the Internet, the importance of multidisciplinary collaboration, and access to scientific knowledge by people who are not health professionals will also be important factors in understanding how research synthesis can have an impact on the health and lives of people throughout the world.

GUIDELINES FOR DESIGNING AND REPORTING BETTER STUDIES

In the late 1990s, health sciences experts began to question the quality of studies reporting randomized controlled trials (RCTs). This concern led eventually to the publication of guidelines about how to design and report studies with RCTs as well as other designs, five of which are described in this section. As with the broader field of research synthesis, the specifics of early guideline development tended to be international in character. The number of guidelines has proliferated since then, and a current listing can be found at the National Guideline Clearinghouse (http://www.guideline.gov).

Most of the guidelines discussed in this section include a description of the guideline development, a checklist for designing and reporting better studies, and a flow chart for tracking the subjects of the study from recruitment to completion of the analysis. These five guidelines focus on studies with either RCTs (randomized clinical/controlled trials) (CONSORT or SPIRIT) or non-RCTs, known in the epidemiological literature as observational studies (cohort, case-control, and cross-sectional studies) (STROBE). Two other kinds of guidelines are for studies of meta-analysis of observational studies (MOOSE), and the validity and reliability of diagnostic measures (STARD).

Although epidemiological designs are most often used in medical or clinical journals, other research designs from the behavioral sciences are also part of the medical literature. Behavioral sciences designs, which are parallel but different from the epidemiological designs, include experimental designs that require randomization of subjects to two or more groups (similar to RCTs), and three other designs without randomization: quasi-experimental, pre-experimental, and observational designs.

Note the difference in the definition of "observational." In epidemiology, observational designs are any of the nonrandomized designs; alternatively, in behavioral sciences designs, "observational" means one specific design that describes the systematic observation and reporting about one group of subjects at one point in time, with no intervention or pretests or posttests. Although the behavioral sciences designs are emphasized in this book, the epidemiological designs are discussed here in terms of the guidelines for the medical or clinical literature. It is important for students in the health sciences to know both systems, epidemiological and behavioral sciences designs.

The following section provides an overview of five selected guidelines for improving the reporting of studies with different methodological designs in the peer-reviewed literature. Of course, improving the reporting of a study depends not only on a specific research question, but also on an appropriate methodological design; thus, these guidelines are also useful in planning such a study.

CONSORT (Consolidated Standards of Reporting Trials)

The CONSORT Statement has two parts: (1) a checklist that describes the basics of what an RCT is and how it is to be reported in a paper submitted to a journal, and (2) a flowchart for tracking the number of patients from eligibility to completion of the trial. The CONSORT Statement has undergone three major revisions. It was published initially in 1996,[47] revised in 2001,[48] and most recently issued in 2010.[49]

The 2010 CONSORT consists of a 25-item checklist and a flowchart documenting the number of subjects assessed for eligibility, randomized to two or more groups with/without intervention, lost to follow-up, and included in the final analysis. The authors urge that the checklist be used together with the companion paper, CONSORT 2010 Explanation and Elaboration, which provides greater detail about the 25 items.[50] The 2010 CONSORT Statement was published simultaneously in several international journals, including Annals of Internal Medicine, British Medical Journal, Lancet, PLoS Medicine, and Journal of Clinical Epidemiology. Over 400 peer-reviewed journals have endorsed the CONSORT Statement and included it in the "Instructions to Authors" section. Updates and future revisions can be obtained at their website (http://www.consort-statement.org).

SPIRIT (Standard Protocol Items: Recommendations for Interventional Trials)

The SPIRIT 2013 Statement for RCTs evolved from several previous international conferences and papers by another group of experts, as described in their paper[51] published simultaneously in the Annals of Internal Medicine and the British Medical Journal. The SPIRIT 2013 Checklist consisted of 33 items for study design, conduct, reporting, and appraisal of randomized clinical or controlled trials. A comparison between the items in the 2013 SPIRIT with 2010 CONSORT checklists shows considerable overlap. Like the CONSORT Statement, authors of the SPIRIT paper have also published a companion article on Explanation and Elaboration about the details of each item.[52] A website for future revisions of the SPIRIT 2013 statement is: http://www.spirit-statement.org.

STROBE (Strengthening the Reporting of Observational Studies in Epidemiology)

The gold standard for clinical research is the RCT; however, most studies in clinical journals are observational, based on cohort, case-control, or cross-sectional designs. Both CONSORT and SPIRIT address RCTs, and STROBE focuses on the other epidemiological designs. The 2007 STROBE Statement[53] describes its development, a 22-item checklist, and a separate publication of explanation and elaboration about the items.[54] Both papers, published simultaneously in the Annals of Internal Medicine, Epidemiology, and PLoS Medicine, are freely accessible and can be downloaded as a PDF on the PLoS Medicine website (http://journals.plos.org/plosmedicine/article?id=10.1371/journal.pmed.0040297).

The STROBE Explanation and Elaboration paper by Vandenbroucke et al.[54] includes both a flowchart for tracking numbers of subjects in a study using these designs and an excellent summary of definitions and differences of the three observational designs (cohort studies, case-control studies, cross-sectional studies). The section on the three observational designs alone should be required reading for all health sciences students. (See Box 1. Main study designs covered by STROBE in the Vandenbroucke et al. paper.) The STROBE website (http://www.strobe-statement.org) lists the journals that include the STROBE statement in their instructions for authors. *At the website, click the tab Endorsement to see the list of journals.*

MOOSE (Meta-Analysis Of Observational Studies in Epidemiology

Standards for reporting MOOSE were developed by an international, multidisciplinary group of experts in a series of workshops sponsored by the Centers for Disease Control in the United States. The MOOSE 2000 paper describes their checklist for authors, editors, and reviewers of these kinds of studies.[55] The checklist consists of 35 items, categorized under six headings: background, search strategy, methods, results, discussion, and conclusions. Under the search strategy, the checklist also includes the reporting of citations located and included in or excluded from the final meta-analysis. Although the checklist was designed for studies that used existing databases for these designs, as noted under Comments, even meta-analyses of RCTs were considered observational studies. Thus, the MOOSE checklist would be applicable to all epidemiological designs. MOOSE is included in the EQUATOR Network (http://www.equator-network.org /reporting-guidelines/meta-analysis-of-observational-studies-in-epidemiology-a -proposal-for-reporting-meta-analysis-of-observational-studies-in-epidemiology -moose-group).

STARD (STAndards for Reporting Diagnostic Accuracy)

Another group of experts became concerned about the quality of reporting the completeness and the transparency of diagnostic accuracy, specifically the ability of readers to determine the potential for bias in a study and generalization of results from the study to a population. The resulting STARD Statement was to be used in conjunction with other guidelines, such as CONSORT, if applicable. Initially published simultaneously in over 20 journals in 2003,[56] the STARD

Statement was recently updated in a 2015 paper published simultaneously in BMJ, Radiology, and Clinical Chemistry.[57] The 2015 checklist consists of 30 items listed under seven categories: title, abstract, introduction, methods, results, discussion, and other information. A flowchart was included to document numbers of subjects as the study progressed. A PDF copy of the 2015 STARD paper is available online (http://www.equator-network.org/wp-content/uploads/2015/03/STARD-2015-paper.pdf). Both the 30-item checklist and the STARD 2015 flow diagram of participants are available online (http://www.equator-network.org/reporting-guidelines/stard). Future updates, revisions, and extensions are also available at this website.

Summary

Five guidelines for designing better studies were described in this section: CONSORT, SPIRIT, STROBE, MOOSE, and STARD. With the exception of the first two (CONSORT and SPIRIT), each of these guidelines serves a different purpose with a specific type of study. This set of five is only the first of many guidelines that have been issued over the years. It is important to remember the following two things about this set compared with the other guidelines introduced later in this chapter: (1) This set is for designing a study with the specific characteristics as stated, for example, if you are reviewing an RCT (or a study with an experimental design), then you will use either the CONSORT or SPIRIT guideline, not one of the others. But if the study is limited to one of the nonrandomized designs, then you will use the STROBE guideline. (2) More importantly, because your goal is to evaluate studies in a literature review, you might wait until you have assembled all of the relevant source documents, then use the appropriate guideline, for example, CONSORT, STROBE, to apply to each of the studies with the specific designs. Now, back to the brief history of research synthesis.

GUIDELINES FOR EXPERT-LED REVIEWS

Gaining a Perspective: A Typology of Reviews

Beginning in 2009, there were further major developments in the field of research synthesis in the health sciences, with strong leadership by scientists and clinicians in the UK. This resulted in different types of guidelines for scientific and clinical papers in the peer-reviewed literature. One of the best ways to gain a perspective on what was happening at the beginning of this period of expansion is to read Grant and Booth's paper about their typology of 14 kinds of reviews.[60] The authors, based respectively in nursing and health and related research in two British universities, describe each type of review, their perceived strengths and weaknesses, and an example from the literature.

Currently, the number of types of reviews exceeds the 14 described by Grant and Booth, but some of the terms have become standardized, such as systematic review, which refers to the application of one or more of the standards for expert-led reviews, such as PRISMA or the IOM Standards, as described in this section. "Standardized Review" is an appropriate keyword to use in PubMed or other databases for finding these types of secondary source documents.

Similarities and Differences Between Two Types of Guidelines

The guidelines in the section above, Guidelines for Designing and Reporting Better Studies, differ from those described in this section, Guidelines for Expert-LED Reviews, by intended audience, purpose of the review, and ways in which the final paper will be used. Similarities and differences between these two types of guidelines are summarized in **Table 1-1**.

For example, the CONSORT Statement is to be used by author(s) in designing, implementing, and reporting a scientific study in a paper submitted for peer-review and by editors/journal reviewers in reviewing that submission for publication, whereas the PRISMA Statement is for an expert-led, multidisciplinary team in designing, administering, and reporting a review of multiple publications about a specific scientific topic. The major differences are in the audience to whom the guideline is addressed (authors/journal reviewers vs. team of expert reviewers), the scope of the review (a single study to be submitted to a peer-reviewed journal vs. evaluation of multiple studies already published in multiple journals), and the ways in which the guideline will be used (assess a single study vs. evaluate a review of multiple studies in a review). What they have in common is a similar format: a statement consisting of a checklist, a flowchart of either subjects (e.g., CONSORT) or documents (e.g., PRISMA), and often a companion paper on the explanation and elaboration of the checklist items.

With this understanding of the similarities and differences between these two categories of guidelines, we turn now to a description of some of the guidelines for expert-led systematic reviews.

Table 1-1 Similarities and Differences Between Guidelines for Designing and Reporting Better Studies and Guidelines for Expert-Led Reviews

Type of Guideline	Audience	Purpose of Guideline	Ways in Which Guideline Will Also Be Used
Guidelines for designing and reporting better studies (CONSORT, SPIRIT, STROBE, MOOSE, STARD)	Authors of scientific papers Journal editors & reviewers of medical/clinical journals	Checklist and flowchart of subjects from eligibility to analysis in the design and report of a peer-reviewed scientific paper Criteria for review for publication of a primary source paper	Description of design & report of scientific paper submitted to journal for publication Review of scientific paper submitted for journal publication
Guidelines for expert-led reviews of publications (PRISMA, IOM Standards, STROBING Review)	Teams of experts in planning, administering, writing, and reporting a scientific paper Journal editors & reviewers of medical/clinical journals	Checklist and flowchart of papers (documents) considered in planning, administering, and reporting of systematic review or meta-analysis Checklist for evaluating report of systematic review or meta-analysis	Checklist and flowchart used in review of systematic review or meta-analysis upon submission for journal publication Checklist and flowchart for evaluating expert-led systematic review or meta-analysis submitted for journal publication

PRISMA, PROSPERO, AND A JOURNAL

PRISMA: A Guideline for Conducting a Systematic Review or Meta-analysis

While recognizing the importance of the Cochrane Collaboration in research synthesis, the scientific field still needed guidelines for groups of experts independent of the Cochrane (although individual members may have such an affiliation), whose purpose was to synthesize peer-reviewed papers in their areas of expertise. This need was addressed in 2009 when the PRISMA Statement was published in the British Medical Journal (BMJ) by authors from Canada, Italy, and the UK. PRISMA had evolved from an earlier set of guidelines, QUORM.[3]

The 2009 PRISMA Statement consists of three parts: (1) a checklist for organizing, planning, and reporting either a systematic review or meta-analysis, (2) a companion paper about the explanation and elaboration of each item in the checklist,[61] and (3) a flow chart for tracking the numbers of records or documents identified, screened for inclusion, eligible, and included in qualitative and quantitative syntheses.

The first published guideline, the 2009 PRISMA Statement, was for studies based on aggregate data. A second guideline, the 2015 PRISMA-IPD, applied to studies that used individual patient data (IPD). In both of these guidelines, the focus was on RCT studies, although this was not a requirement, as well as those with qualitative and quantitative data.[62] The authors cautioned that the 2009 PRISMA checklist was not to be used to assess the quality of a systematic review. Over the years, additional PRISMA guidelines have been published as extensions. The checklists for PRISMA, PRISMA-IPD, and other extensions are available online (http://www.prisma-statement.org). This website also provides the PRISMA Flowchart for Tracking Source Documents Throughout the Review Process and is shown in **Exhibit 1-1**.

PRISMA Flowchart and the Matrix Method

The use of the PRISMA Flowchart[3] is rapidly becoming a standard in any review of the literature because of its innovative and efficient design. For that reason, the PRISMA Flowchart[3] is now an important addition to be used with the Matrix Method. But the PRISMA Flowchart[3] is the only component of the PRISMA Statement that should be used in your review. The other two components, the 27-item PRISMA Checklist[3] and the explanation and elaboration of each item

EXHIBIT 1-1   PRISMA Flowchart for Tracking Source Documents Throughout the Review Process

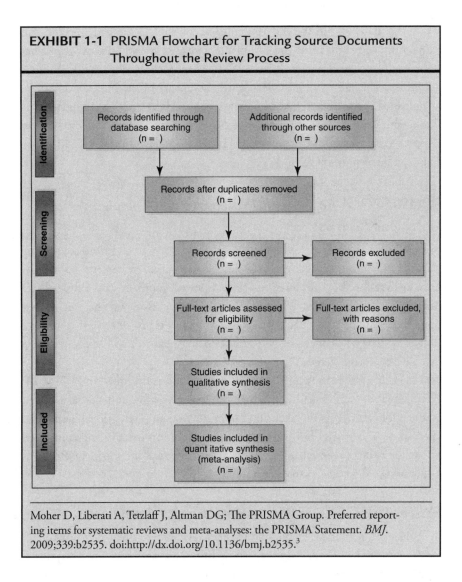

Moher D, Liberati A, Tetzlaff J, Altman DG; The PRISMA Group. Preferred reporting items for systematic reviews and meta-analyses: the PRISMA Statement. *BMJ.* 2009;339:b2535. doi:http://dx.doi.org/10.1136/bmj.b2535.[3]

in the checklist,[61] are intended for expert-led teams in conducting systematic reviews or meta-analyses.

In using the PRISMA Flowchart[3] in your review of the literature, you must provide a citation every time you use it or refer to it. Here are the terms by the authors of the PRISMA Statement[3] for using the flowchart in your own work:

See this statement in the BMJ publication[3] by Moher, Liberati, Tetzlaff, and Altman under Footnotes at the end of the paper. At the website, www.prisma-statement.org, there is a copy of the PRISMA Flowchart described as the PRISMA 2009 Flow Diagram[3] in the upper-right-hand corner of the screen that can be downloaded and modified by adding your own tracking numbers of documents throughout your review of the literature. More about the PRISMA Flowchart[3] in Chapter 4, and again in Chapter 6 of this book. A copy of the PRISMA Flowchart can be seen in Exhibit 1-1.

PROSPERO: A Registry for Prospective and Completed Systematic Reviews

In order to create a more efficient system for experts in the time-consuming tasks of organizing, preparing, analyzing, and writing systematic reviews or meta-analyses to be submitted to peer-reviewed journals, the PROSPERO Registry was launched in 2012 by the Center for Reviews and Dissemination, University of York, UK.[63] The Registry invites teams of experts to register systematic reviews or meta-analysis studies being planned, and publishes those that have been completed.

A checklist for creating a PROSPERO proposal was described in PRISMA-P (PRISMA-Protocols) issued in 2015.[64] The Registry is free and can be accessed by the public as well as the scientific community on an international basis, with open access and articles freely available online. Both prospective and completed systematic reviews are available in this Registry. The website for PROSPERO is http://www.crd.york.ac.uk/prospero.

SYSTEMATIC REVIEWS: A Peer-Reviewed Journal

In 2012, the first issue of an online, peer-reviewed journal, SYSTEMATIC REVIEWS, was launched.[65] Their website is: http://www.systematicreviewsjournal .com. Their commitment to an international mission can be seen in the affiliations of the three editors-in-chief: the Ottawa Hospital Research Institute, University of Ottawa, Canada; the RAND Corporation and UCLA School of Medicine, USA; and the Centre for Reviews and Dissemination, University of York, UK.

With the creation of this journal, an infrastructure for independent teams of reviewers was complete: (1) a set of guidelines, PRISMA,[3] providing expert teams in the field with a checklist of how a systematic review or meta-analysis can be administered and what to include, (2) a registry, PROSPERO,[63] to avoid overlapping efforts by experts in the field interested in conducting systematic reviews intended for publication as well as a list of completed reviews, and (3) an electronic, peer-reviewed, open access journal, SYSTEMATIC REVIEWS,[65] as one of several international journals available in the field for publishing the reviews. All three elements of this infrastructure have since been used throughout the world by researchers and specialists in clinical fields, including those in the United States, since 2012.

IOM STANDARDS FOR SYSTEMATIC REVIEWS: FINDING WHAT WORKS IN HEALTH CARE

In the United States, the IOM, a division of the National Academies of Sciences, Engineering, and Medicine, issued their own standards in 2011 for initiating and reporting a systematic review, comparable to the PRISMA Statement. These IOM Standards for Systematic Reviews can be found at their website (http://iom .nationalacademies.org/Reports/2011/Finding-What-Works-in-Health-Care -Standards-for-Systematic-Reviews.aspx; *in the box labeled Report at a Glance, click on Standards for Systematic Reviews*). The IOM Standards were developed for studies that addressed evidence- based practice issues and to guide decisions about health care in the United States under the Affordable Care Act after its implementation in 2013.

The 21 IOM standards, like the 27 items in the PRISMA Checklist,[3] are comprehensive and clearly focused on systematic reviews by multidisciplinary teams of experts, with funding and staff to prepare each review for publication in a peer-reviewed journal. At the IOM website, standards are described for (1) initiating a systematic review, (2) finding and assessing individual studies, (3) synthesizing the body of evidence, and (4) reporting systematic reviews. Reading through the standards can be of use to those who are learning how to prepare a plan for a literature review, but too many of the items in the checklist are well beyond the level of understanding of the beginning reviewer; thus the goal of conducting a systematic review or meta-analysis is more appropriate to teams of highly experienced reviewers preparing systematic reviews.

SCOPING REVIEWS: FINDING THE GAPS IN EXISTING LITERATURE

A scoping review is a rigorously defined protocol used to identify the gaps in research on a specific subject. In general, the topic being reviewed has not fully matured to justify a systematic review or meta-analysis, but is of importance to healthcare policy and other health sciences research in its earlier stages. For example, a study of the first report in the United States of AIDS, in 1981, described only five subjects. This was an observational design, based on careful review and description of the case histories; there was no comparison group, only careful observation.[66] Over the following decade, approximately 400 reports were reported with increasingly sophisticated methods and research questions about the disease.[67] Thus in the early 1980s, the AIDS literature did not have a sufficient number of papers to warrant a systematic review, but the literature could qualify for a scoping review.

The 2005 paper by Arksey and O'Malley was one of the first to describe a methodological framework for conducting scoping studies.[68] There was a problem with the Arksey and O'Malley paper, however, caused by a significant delay between the year the manuscript was accepted (2003) and its publication (2005). None of the papers in the references section is newer than 2002. Nonetheless, the Arksey and O'Malley paper is often the classic starting point in describing the history of scoping reviews.

A more specialized focus was a review of scoping studies in the nursing literature in 2009,[69] which still found problems with the existing methodology. In 2010, Levac et al. described improvements to the Arksey and O'Malley methodology and upgraded the quality of this type of review.[70] The practicalities of implementing both the Arksey and O'Malley framework and the Levac modifications were described by a large interprofessional group of experts in a 2013 paper, including their suggestions for working together as a team.[71]

Perhaps it was inevitable that a paper was published recently (2014) of a scoping review of scoping reviews in which the authors further documented the need for improving the methodology.[72] Finally, the Joanna Briggs Institute (JBI) at the University of Adelaide, South Australia, AU, published an online guide, "Reviewers' Manual 2015: Methodology for JBI Scoping Reviews," that offers a detailed set of instructions for this type of expert-led review, available at their website (http://joannabriggs.org/assets/docs/sumari/Reviewers-Manual_Methodology-for-JBI-Scoping-Reviews_2015_v2.pdf). These five papers plus the manual provide an excellent overview of the methodology and application of scoping reviews up to 2015 for those interested in using this approach.

FUTURE GUIDELINES AND REVISIONS IN THE HEALTH SCIENCES LITERATURE

As shown in this summary, many guidelines are updated every few years, often in response to rapid changes in the clinical or scientific fields. This section includes three sources for staying up to date about new guidelines and systematic reviews or meta-analyses that have been updated and revised. These sources are like three tools in your scientific repertoire as you review the literature: not necessarily used every day, but good to know about.

Hint

For the first two of the three sources in this section, collaborate with a partner and use a computer. Have the partner read aloud the instructions in italics, and you apply them on the computer. (For example, go to the National Guideline Clearinghouse website (www .guideline.gov), and do just what the instructions say.) Then reverse roles. Explore the website together to see what else you can learn.

This will be time well spent when you get into creating your own review of the literature. (If you do not team up with someone, then it is like reading the instructions for how to ride a bicycle the first time you do it, with no bicycle and no other person to help you. Sure, you can do it by yourself, but it is not nearly as much fun!)

National Guideline Clearinghouse (NGC): An On-Going Source of Guidelines

The National Guideline Clearinghouse (NGC) was launched in 1999 by the Agency for Health Research (AHRQ), a U.S. government agency, as described at this website: http://www.guideline.gov. A categorization of guidelines by disease/ condition, treatment/intervention, and health services administration is available. (*At the website, go to the box to the left, click Guidelines, then under Browse, click By Topic. Clicking the arrow next to the topic provides further classification of the guidelines.*) Clinical practice guidelines are restricted to only those submitted or revised within the past 5 years.

Further information about specific guidelines by clinical specialty is provided under another tab. (At the website in the box to the left, pull down the tab Guideline Matrix, which describes Clinical Specialty by Methods Used to Analyze the Evidence. Each cell in this matrix has the number of guidelines in the database, and clicking that number will provide each citation and the NGC number.) This is an invaluable tool. For example, if you want to review all guidelines for Nursing that had a Systematic Review with Evidence Tables, then do this: Click Guideline Matrix, go down to "Nursing," scroll the matrix over to the last column on the right with the title "Methods Used to Analyze the Evidence." Click the number in the cell to go to a complete list of the citations for all guidelines currently available. Scroll down that list to select which guideline you are interested in.

To see each of the guidelines in greater detail, expand the tab Guideline Syntheses. Alternatively, go to the tab FAQ for further information about the development of the guidelines. The NGC is updated weekly at a website that is free, available to the public, and accessible from a general browser. AHRQ has produced a YouTube tutorial about the Search and Browse features of the NGC, which you can access by typing this into your browser: National Guideline Clearinghouse: Search & Browse (Official Tutorial).

The number of guidelines at http://www.guideline.gov can be daunting, with over 2,000 listed in 2015. (At the Home Page, under the Guidelines tab, under Browse, click Guideline Index to see a current count of individual guideline summaries in the database.) There are ways to narrow your search for specific guidelines. Use the Search box at the top of each page, or click the FAQ tab to see commonly asked questions and answers.

The website also lists guidelines added within the past 2 weeks: *from the Home page, go to Guidelines tab, under Browse, click Guidelines in Progress.* A current list of guidelines that have been either updated or withdrawn in the NGC Archive is available. *(Under the Guidelines tab, under the Browse section, click Guideline Archive for guidelines that have been either Updated or Withdrawn. Both updated/ withdrawn lists include a citation for each guideline.)*

EQUATOR Network: Enhancing the Quality and Transparency of Health Research

Another way of tracking guidelines is to examine reviews by study type, for example, randomized trials, systematic reviews, qualitative research, available at the EQUATOR Network website: http://www.equator-network.org. The mission of this international umbrella organization is to provide a reliable source for improving the reporting of health research studies with the goal of supporting research reproducibility and usefulness (http://www.equator-network.org/about -us/equatornewor-what-we-do-and-how-we-are-organized).

The EQUATOR Network grew out of an international project begun in 2006 at Oxford, UK, and now has three centres based in the UK, France, and Canada. In addition to current events and announcements of international meetings, the EQUATOR Network succinctly summarizes types of reporting guidelines, such as CONSORT and PRISMA.

The website is free and includes both guidelines completed since 1996, and guidelines under development. (Under "Library for health research reporting" on the Home page, click "Reporting guidelines under development" for a list of guidelines currently under development.) Currently (late 2015), the list includes 284 completed guidelines and is growing. The website also lists courses and events, news, a blog, and other information about guidelines and their development.

LIVING SYSTEMATIC REVIEWS: A Perpetual Source

Despite the intense effort needed to organize and complete a systematic review or meta-analysis, once published, its usefulness is limited to an estimated 2.5–5.5 years, mainly because of rapid developments in the field.[73] This time limitation is related to the broader issue of a gap between research and healthcare practice. To address both of these problems, a new term, LIVING SYSTEMATIC REVIEW, has been created to describe an online update or revision of a systematic review or meta-analysis that takes into account new research or subsequent developments in the field. This concept and its practice are quickly evolving, and publications about LIVING SYSTEMATIC REVIEWS can probably best be found through Google Scholar or Google at this point in time.[74]

DIFFERENCES BETWEEN SYSTEMATIC REVIEWS, SCOPING REVIEWS, AND REVIEWS OF THE LITERATURE

Systematic Reviews

A systematic review requires a clear and concise question; uses systematic and explicit methods to identify, select, and critically evaluate relevant research; and collects and analyzes data from authors of such documents as part of the review process.[75] Both a systematic review and a review of the literature use primary source data such as peer-reviewed papers about a study, although PRISMA guidelines also permit documents from other sources, such as the grey literature or editorials. One of the major differences is that the PRISMA Statement[3] assumes that the reviewers are experts in their fields, such as clinical sciences, research design, methodology, and biostatistics, and have funding for staff and other resources for a systematic review; whereas a review of the literature assumes an individual, usually a graduate/professional student, who is conducting and completing an original study with minimal funding for resources. The product of a systematic review is either a narrative synthesis of the research or a meta-analysis if sufficient numbers of studies permit, or both (usually in a mixed mode review). A narrative synthesis consists of a nonstatistical summary of the literature, in contrast to a meta-analysis review of the literature.

Scoping Reviews

A Scoping Review may be appropriate for review studies that do not have enough peer-reviewed papers to permit a PRISMA review.[3] But systematic reviews, scoping reviews, and a review of the literature using the Matrix Method share in the rigor in which the studies are evaluated by reading, selecting, analyzing and reporting the results. All three of these types of reviews require attention to standardization of research synthesis methods. And, in all three types of reviews, there is a commitment to the reproducibility and replication of the methods in selecting and excluding source documents. This is accomplished with the use of a flowchart[3] for tracking the numbers of source documents through the different stages of the review process.

Reviews of the Literature: The Matrix Method

As described in this book, a review of the literature consists of a structured process for defining the research question, selecting, reading, organizing, analyzing, and writing a narrative synthesis of previous research on a topic of interest to the beginning graduate or professional student in the health sciences. The Matrix Method is intended to teach you how to read a paper, organize the review using the Matrix Method, analyze it, and create a narrative synthesis. The alternative, a meta-analysis, is not taught in this book (other than to describe it) and is beyond the scope of what is expected of a beginning student.

Unlike the expert-led reviews, this review of the literature is envisioned as a solo activity, with guidance by faculty or mentors. The emphasis is on primary source documents, preferably in the peer-reviewed literature, with possibly a section on secondary source reviews (such as systematic reviews) or tertiary reviews (such as reviews of reviews). A review of the literature is the fundamental first step in how to read and analyze papers by other scientists and determine what is missing in this body of work. Thus, a review of the literature, as described in this book, is the initial step for the student's proposal for an independent scientific study, usually in the form of a Master's project or doctoral dissertation. With this perspective about research synthesis, we now turn to an introduction and overview of the Matrix Method for reviewing the literature.

THE MATRIX METHOD: DEFINITION AND OVERVIEW

The surfeit of information in the health sciences literature presents both a problem and an opportunity. What is needed is a structured way of organizing and conducting a literature review. The Matrix Method offers one such system. With this section of Chapter 1, we now get down to the details of "how to do it." What follows is a summary of those details.

The Matrix Method is both a structure and a process for reviewing the literature. The structure is provided by the Master Folder that contains all of the notes and documentations you accumulated as you reviewed the literature. The Master Folder includes four major subfolders, as shown in **Exhibit 1-2**, consisting of the following:

1. Paper Trail Folder—documenting your search of the literature: This is a record of the search process you used to identify relevant materials. Examples include which librarians or other experts you talked to about the search, notes about the materials examined, keywords used to search the electronic bibliographic databases, and, especially, a list of instructions for electronic searches and the instructions you gave. Think of this as a

EXHIBIT 1-2 Structure of the Matrix Method: Subfolders in the Master Folder	
Type of Subfolder	**Purpose**
• Paper Trail Folder	Documenting your search of the literature
• Documents Folder	Storing documents for review
• Review Matrix Folder	Abstracting each document using the Matrix Method
• Synthesis Folder	Writing the review of the literature

chronological diary or personal blog about the process you went through as you conducted this review of the literature.

It is here in the Paper Trail Folder that you will begin to build the PRISMA Flowchart of Documents[3] that you will eventually report in your final paper. More about this in Chapter 4.

2. Documents Folder—organizing documents for review: This section includes a downloaded copy, PDF file, or link to the journal articles, book chapters, and other materials gathered for your review of the literature. These are the documents used to create a review matrix, which goes in the third folder.

3. Review Matrix Folder—abstracting each document: The review matrix is a spreadsheet or table with columns and rows that you use to abstract selected information about each journal article, book chapter, or other materials included in your review of the literature.

4. Synthesis Folder—writing the review of the literature: This is the outcome of your use of the Matrix Method, a written synthesis of your critical review of the literature based on the materials you abstracted in the review matrix. The Synthesis will include your narrative review of the literature and a copy of the most recent number of documents you identified at each stage in the PRISMA Flowchart of Information Through Defined Phases of this Literature Review. [3]

In addition to structure in the form of a Master Folder, the Matrix Method also provides a process for how to create and use the materials in each of the four folders. The Matrix Method was specifically designed for reviews of the health sciences literature, but it can be used for reviews of the literature in any field by anyone at any level of expertise, from novice to seasoned reviewer. The key to the versatility of the Matrix Method lies in the use of the review matrix, which is described briefly here.

REVIEW MATRIX: A VERSATILE TOOL

With a review matrix, you create a structured abstract of all the source documents from your literature review. A review matrix is like a spreadsheet or a table—a rectangular arrangement of columns and rows. All that is needed to set up a blank review matrix is a blank spreadsheet or the table option in a word processor.

The columns across the top of a review matrix are the topics or headings you use to abstract each document or study. The rows down the page are the

EXHIBIT 1-3 Example of the Format of a Review Matrix			
Column 1	**Column 2**	**Column 3**	**Column 4**
Example: **Author, title, journal**	Example: **Year**	Example: **Purpose**	Example: **Type of study design**
Row 1 Journal article 1	1995	Drug treatment for epilepsy	Experimental study
Row 2 Journal article 2	1997	Drug treatment	Case-control study for depression

documents or studies. The point at which each column and row meets is a cell, which is where you write notes about a document. An example of the format for a review matrix is shown in **Exhibit 1-3**, in which there are four columns and two rows. Each column has a topic—such as author/title/journal, year, purpose, or type of study design—and each row consists of a journal article. Thus, the review matrix is a place to record notes about each article, paper, study, or report on the basis of a standard set of column topics.

Column topics can range from very general to specific. For example, a review matrix for Shakespeare's plays might include these column topics: setting, characters, chief protagonist, chief antagonist, and psychological theme. Alternatively, if the focus was on the scientific literature, the matrix would feature other kinds of column topics: hypothesis, independent variables, dependent variable, methodological design, and sampling design.

No matter what the level of expertise or area of focus is, you are entirely in control of the review matrix. You decide which column topics to use and which documents or studies to review. The process you use to make those decisions— which topics, which documents—is described in this text. In the course of making those decisions, abstracting the articles, and writing the synthesis, you begin to take ownership of the literature.

OVERVIEW OF CHAPTERS AND APPENDICES

The creation and use of the review matrix and Master Folder are described in the remaining chapters. Although the Matrix Method can be applied to the literature on just about any topic, there is an emphasis throughout this text on the health sciences. The nine chapters in this text are organized into the following three parts:

- Part I. Fundamentals of a Literature Review—Chapters 1 and 2
- Part II. The Matrix Method—Chapters 3 through 6
- Part III. Applications Using the Matrix Method—Chapters 7 through 9

Chapters 2 through 9 are described briefly here, followed by an overview of the Appendices. At the end of each chapter is a section titled "Caroline's Quest," which includes practical examples of how the concepts can be applied.

Chapter 2: Basic Concepts

This chapter consists of definitions of concepts that are fundamental in any review of the literature, especially those used in the Matrix Method. Also included in this chapter is a description of the different parts of a typical scientific paper published in most health-related journals. If you know where to find specific topics, then you will be in a better position to abstract the study. Chapter 2 also describes the basic elements of a methodological review of the literature. These elements can be used as the sole basis of a review or, more realistically, as a list of possibilities for inclusion, together with the content of the paper under review. A list of potential column topics for reviewing the research methodology in the scientific literature is given in the section "A Methodological Review of the Literature: The Methods Map."

Chapter 3: Paper Trail Folder: How to Plan and Manage a Search of the Literature

This chapter describes what steps to take in doing a review of the literature, how to develop a keywords list, how to locate source materials; how to use the snowballing technique; what to consider in a computer search of established databases such as MEDLINE, PsycINFO, and Science Citation Index; and use of the Internet.

Chapter 4: Documents Folder: How to Select and Organize Documents for Review

This chapter includes a description of how to choose documents and organize journal articles and other source materials. The advantages of maintaining a chronologically ordered set of PDF files or other types of electronic copies in the Documents Folder are also discussed.

Chapter 5: Review Matrix Folder: How to Abstract the Research Literature

The review matrix is the heart of the Matrix Method. This chapter describes how to set up a review matrix, including issues such as choosing topics to abstract, variations in topics, addition of topics later in the process, and a step-by-step guide for constructing the review matrix.

Chapter 6: Synthesis Folder: How to Use a Review Matrix to Write a Synthesis

This chapter is a description of how to use the review matrix to critically analyze and write a narrative review of the literature, including a discussion of the differences between a summary and a synthesis. The importance of tracking the number of source documents and including them in the PRISMA Flowchart[3] is emphasized in this chapter. Your adaptation of the PRISMA Flowchart[3] will be included in your final copy of your narrative synthesis in the Synthesis Folder.

Chapter 7: A Library of Master Folders

This chapter describes the advantages of maintaining a collection of Master Folders for use over time, or by a team of people, or across interrelated topics. Specifics include how to create and expand a library of Master Folders.

Chapter 8: The Matrix Indexing System

This chapter describes a system for integrating information from electronic databases and reference libraries created with reference management software and copies of papers in the Documents Folder in the Master Folder. The advantages of this system are discussed, together with information on how to set up and use such a system.

Chapter 9: Matrix Applications by Health Sciences Professionals

This chapter describes four kinds of applications for the experienced health sciences professional. These include the use of the Matrix Method in (1) conducting a research project, from writing a grant proposal to publishing the results; (2) standardizing the review process for a meta-analysis; (3) creating and using clinical practice guidelines; and (4) applying the concepts of evidence-based medicine.

Appendix A: Useful Resources for Literature Reviews

This is a handy list of books, journals, and Internet websites that can be useful when searching for scientific literature that is not available in the standard sources. The appendix is a potpourri of useful information.

Appendix B: Structure of Computer Folders for the Matrix Method

This appendix describes how to create and organize computer folders on your desktop for the Matrix Method. Examples are given to help you understand this structure before you use the Matrix Method to review the literature.

Appendix C: Data Visualization: A Digital Exploration

This appendix describes recent advances in data visualization and how these resources could be used in describing scientific research. In this appendix, you go into a digital environment and explore the possibilities for the use of data visualization for a review of the literature now and in the future. Check the front cover of this book to obtain your password that gives you access to Appendix C.

REFERENCES TO WEBSITES

Website addresses are given throughout the remaining chapters, and especially in Appendix A. Each address on the Internet, called a universal resource locator (URL), was examined and determined to be accurate and functional at the time this text was published; however, the Internet is a dynamic environment, and URLs can change on an hourly basis. For this reason, neither the author nor the publisher is responsible for the accuracy of the URLs provided in this text.

Caroline's Quest: Understanding the Process

Just as a picture can be worth a thousand words in explaining a concept, a practical example can be equally valuable in demonstrating the process of using a strategy such as the Matrix Method. With that in mind, each of the nine chapters in this book will conclude with a description of the experiences of a typical graduate student, Caroline Collins, as she learns about matrix applications.

Caroline Collins is learning how to use the Matrix Method and the Matrix Indexing System to review the literature on smoking behavior for her master's thesis in public health. Caroline's thesis topic is the characteristics of teenage girls who smoke.

Caroline tends to be a bit impatient and will occasionally try to take shortcuts to avoid some of the more time-consuming details of the Matrix Method. Fortunately, she meets weekly with her advisor, Professor Dickerson, who gives her advice about using the matrix applications. Caroline's experiences and Professor Dickerson's explanations illustrate not only the process but also why certain steps in the Matrix Method are needed and how the Matrix Indexing System can help her organize her materials.

In medieval times, a quest was a chivalrous enterprise involving an adventurous journey that often required courage or determination. In modern times, a quest is defined as a search or pursuit. Although Caroline does not have to deal with dragons in the library, her review of the literature does require persistence and determination in her pursuit of knowledge—a pursuit that is occasionally adventurous. Thus, in both the modern and the ancient senses of the word, Caroline has embarked upon a quest.

A word of advice: If you are having trouble understanding some of the basic problems in implementing the Matrix Method or why certain steps were included, Caroline's adventures will be a valuable resource. All of her questions and objections are based on feedback from my own graduate students over many years, and you may find your own questions here.

What You Should Know or Be Able to Do by the End of This Chapter

A final section about what you have learned will be included at the end of each of Chapters 1 through 6 that describe the Matrix Method. At the end of Chapter 1, you should know or be able to do the following:

1. Define the basic terms about a review of the literature:
   - review of the literature
   - scientific literature
   - source document
   - bibliographic database
   - research synthesis
   - scoping review

2. What does "to own the literature" mean, and how can it be acquired?
3. Describe a brief historical summary of the field of research synthesis.
4. What is a meta-analysis, and how does it differ from a narrative review of the literature?
5. Describe the differences between PRISMA, PROSPERO, and SYSTEMATIC REVIEWS.
6. Describe the PRISMA Statement and the IOM Standards for Systematic Review. How do they compare?
7. What is the difference between the PRISMA Checklist and the PRISMA FLOWCHART for DOCUMENTS?
8. Describe the three sources that you can use to stay up to date about changing guidelines in the future.
9. What is the Matrix Method?
10. What are the four folders in the Master Folder?

REFERENCES

1. Russell CL. An overview of the integrative research review. *Prog Transplant*. 2005; 15(1):8-13.
2. Oxman AD, Cook DJ, Guyatt GH; for the Evidence-Based Medicine Working Group. Users' guides to evidence-based medicine. How to use an overview. *JAMA*. 1994; 272(17):1367-1371.
3. Moher D, Liberati A, Tetzlaff J, Altman DG; The PRISMA Group. Preferred reporting items for systematic reviews and meta-analyses: the PRISMA Statement. *BMJ*. 2009;339:b2535. doi:http://dx.doi.org/10.1136/bmj.b2535.
4. Institute of Medicine. Finding what works in health care: standards for systematic reviews. http://iom.nationalacademies.org/Reports/2011/Finding-What-Works-in -Health-Care-Standards-for-Systematic-Reviews.aspx.
5. National Library of Medicine. *Images from the History of the Public Health Service: Biomedical Research*. U.S. Department of Health and Human Services, Public Health Service; 2005. http://www.nlm.nih.gov/exhibition/phs_history/beginningsbio.html. Accessed January 22, 2013.
6. Institute for Scientific Information. Science citation index 1945–1954: cumulative comparative statistical summary. In: *SCI Science Citation Index Ten Year Cumulation 1945–1954: Guide and Lists of Source Publications*. Vol 8. Philadelphia, PA: Institute for Scientific Information; 1988:18-19.
7. Institute for Scientific Information. Comparative statistical summary 1955–1996. In: *SCI Science Citation Index 1996 Annual Guide and Lists of Source Publications*. Vol 1. Philadelphia, PA: Institute for Scientific Information; 1997:57-63.
8. National Institutes of Health. *NIH Almanac 1997*. Washington, DC: National Institutes of Health; 1997. NIH Publication No. 97-5.
9. Garfield E. In truth, the "flood" of scientific literature is only a myth. *Scientist*. 1991; 5:11-25.

10. Huth EJ. The information explosion. *Bull NY Acad Med.* 1989;65:647-661.

11. Garfield E. Science Citation Index. *Science Citation Index.* 1961, 1, p.v-xvi, 1963. http://garfield.library.upenn.edu/papers/80.pdf. Accessed January 22, 2013.

12. Glass G. Primary, secondary, and meta-analysis of research. *Educ Res.* 1976;5:3-8.

13. Fields MJ, Lohr N, eds. *Guidelines for Clinical Practice: From Development to Use.* Washington, DC: Institute of Medicine, Division of Health Care Services; 1992.

14. Guyatt GH, Rennie D. Users' guides to the medical literature. *JAMA.* 1993;270: 2096-2097.

15. Oxman AD, Sackett DL, Guyatt GH. Users' guides to the medical literature. I. How to get started. *JAMA.* 1993;270:2093-2095.

16. Guyatt GH, Sackett DL, Cook DJ; for the Evidence-Based Medicine Working Group. Users' guides to the medical literature. II. How to use an article about therapy or prevention. A. Are the results of the study valid? *JAMA.* 1993;270:2598-2601.

17. Guyatt GH, Sackett DL, Cook DJ; for the Evidence-Based Medicine Working Group. Users' guides to the medical literature. II. How to use an article about therapy or prevention. B. What were the results and will they help me in caring for my patients? *JAMA.* 1994;271:59-63.

18. Jaeschke R, Guyatt GH, Sackett DL; for the Evidence-Based Medicine Working Group. Users' guides to the medical literature. III. How to use an article about a diagnostic test. B. What are the results and will they help me in caring for my patients? *JAMA.* 1994;271:703-707.

19. Jaeschke R, Guyatt G, Sackett DL; for the Evidence-Based Medicine Working Group. Users' guides to the medical literature. III. How to use an article about a diagnostic test. A. Are the results of the study valid? *JAMA.* 1994;271:389-391.

20. Laupacis A, Wells G, Richardson WS, Tugwell P; for the Evidence-Based Medicine Working Group. Users' guides to the medical literature. V. How to use an article about prognosis. *JAMA.* 1994;272:234-237.

21. Levine M, Walter S, Lee H, Haines T, Holbrook A, Moyer V. Users' guides to the medical literature. IV. How to use an article about harm. *JAMA.* 1994;271:1615-1619.

22. Oxman AD, Cook DJ, Guyatt GH; for the Evidence-Based Medicine Working Group. Users' guides to the medical literature. VI. How to use an overview. *JAMA.* 1994;272:1367-1371.

23. Guyatt GH, Sackett DL, Sinclair JC, Hayward R, Cook DJ, Cook RJ. Users' guides to the medical literature. IX. A method for grading health care recommendations. *JAMA.* 1995;274:1800-1804.

24. Hayward RS, Wilson MC, Tunis SR, Bass EB, Guyatt G; for the Evidence-Based Medicine Working Group. Users' guides to the medical literature. VIII. How to use clinical practice guidelines. A. Are the recommendations valid? *JAMA.* 1995;274:570-574.

25. Richardson WS, Detsky AS; for the Evidence-Based Medicine Working Group. Users' guides to the medical literature. VII. How to use a clinical decision analysis. B. What are the results and will they help me in caring for my patients? *JAMA.* 1995;273: 1610-1613.

26. Richardson WS, Detsky AS; for the Evidence-Based Medicine Working Group. Users' guides to the medical literature. VII. How to use a clinical decision analysis. A. Are the results of the study valid? *JAMA.* 1995;273:1292-1295.

27. Wilson MC, Hayward RS, Tunis SR, Bass EB, Guyatt G; for the Evidence-Based Medicine Working Group. Users' guides to the medical literature. VIII. How to use clinical practice guidelines. B. What are the recommendations and will they help you in caring for your patients? *JAMA.* 1995;274:1630-1632.

28. Naylor CD, Guyatt GH; for the Evidence-Based Medicine Working Group. Users' guides to the medical literature. XI. How to use an article about a clinical utilization review. *JAMA*. 1996;275:1435-1439.

29. Naylor CD, Guyatt GH; for the Evidence-Based Medicine Working Group. Users' guides to the medical literature. X. How to use an article reporting variations in the outcomes of health services. *JAMA*. 1996;275:554-558.

30. Drummond MG, Richardson WS, O'Brien BJ, Levine M, Heyland D; for the Evidence-Based Medicine Working Group. Users' guides to the medical literature. XIII. How to use an article on economic analysis of clinical practice. A. Are the results of the study valid? *JAMA*. 1997;277:1552-1557.

31. Guyatt GH, Naylor CD, Juniper E, et al. Users' guides to the medical literature. XII. How to use articles about health-related quality of life. *JAMA*. 1997;277:1232-1237.

32. O'Brien BJ, Heyland D, Richardson WS, Heyland DK, Jaeschke R, Cook DJ; for the Evidence-Based Medicine Working Group. Users' guides to the medical literature. XIII. How to use an article on economic analysis of clinical practice. B. What are the results and will they help me in caring for my patients? *JAMA*. 1997;277:1802-1806.

33. Dans AL, Dans LF, Guyatt GH, Richardson S; for the Evidence-Based Medicine Working Group. Users' guides to the medical literature. XIV. How to decide on the applicability of clinical trial results to your patient. *JAMA*. 1998;279:545-549.

34. Barratt A, Irwig L, Glasziou P, et al. Users' guides to the medical literature. XVII. How to use guidelines and recommendations about screening. *JAMA*. 1999;281:2029-2034.

35. Bucher H, Guyatt G, Cook D, Holbrook A, McAlister FA; for the Evidence-Based Medicine Working Group. Users' guides to the medical literature. XIX. Applying clinical trial results. A. How to use an article measuring the effect of an intervention on surrogate end points. *JAMA*. 1999;282:771-778.

36. Guyatt G, Sinclair J, Cook D, Glasziou P; for the Evidence-Based Medicine Working Group and the Cochrane Applicability Methods Working Group. Users' guides to the medical literature. XVI. How to use a treatment recommendation. *JAMA*. 1999;281:1836-1843.

37. McAlister F, Laupacis A, Wells G, Sackett DL; for the Evidence-Based Medicine Working Group. Users' guides to the medical literature. XIX. Applying clinical trial results. B. Guidelines for determining whether a drug is exerting (more than) a class effect. *JAMA*. 1999;282:1371-1377.

38. Randolph AG, Haynes RB, Wyatt JC, Cook DJ, Guyatt GH; for the Evidence-Based Medicine Working Group. Users' guides to the medical literature. XVIII. How to use an article evaluating the clinical impact of a computer-based clinical decision support system. *JAMA*. 1999;282:67-74.

39. Richardson WS, Wilson MC, Guyatt GH, Cook DJ, Nishikawa J; for the Evidence-Based Medicine Working Group. Users' guides to the medical literature. XV. How to use an article about disease probability for differential diagnosis. *JAMA*. 1999;281:1214-1219.

40. Giacomini MK, Cook DJ; for the Evidence-Based Medicine Working Group. Users' guides to the medical literature. XXIII. Qualitative research in health care. B. What are the results and how do they help me care for my patients? *JAMA*. 2000;284:478-482.

41. Giacomini M, Cook D; for the Evidence-Based Medicine Working Group. Users' guides to the medical literature. XXIII. Qualitative research in health care. A. Are the results of the study valid? *JAMA*. 2000;284:357-362.

42. Guyatt GH, Haynes RB, Jaeschke RZ, et al. Users' guides to the medical literature. XXV. Evidence-based medicine: principles for applying the users' guides to patient care. *JAMA*. 2000;284:1290-1296.

43. Hunt D, Jaeschke R, McKibbon K; for the Evidence-Based Medicine Working Group. Users' guides to the medical literature. XXI. Using electronic health information resources in evidence-based practice. *JAMA.* 2000;283:1875-1879.

44. McAlister F, Straus S, Guyatt G, Haynes RB; for the Evidence-Based Medicine Working Group. Users' guides to the medical literature. XX. Integrating research evidence with the care of the individual patient. *JAMA.* 2000;283:2829-2836.

45. McGinn T, Guyatt G, Wyer P, Naylor CD, Stiell IG, Richardson WS. Users' guides to the medical literature. XXII. How to use articles about clinical decision rules. *JAMA.* 2000;284:79-84.

46. Richardson WS, Wilson MC, Williams JW Jr, Moyer VA, Naylor CD; for the Evidence-Based Medicine Working Group. Users' guides to the medical literature. XXIV. How to use an article on the clinical manifestations of disease. *JAMA.* 2000;284:869-875.

47. Begg CB, Cho MK, Eastwood S, et al. Improving the quality of reporting of randomized controlled trials: the CONSORT statement. *JAMA.* 1996;276:637-639.

48. Moher D, Schulz KF, Altman D. The CONSORT statement: revised recommendations for improving the quality of reports of parallel-group randomized trials. *JAMA.* 2001;285(15):1987-1991.

49. Schulz KF, Altman DG, Moher D. Consort 2010 statement: updated guidelines for reporting parallel group randomized trials. *Ann Intern Med.* 2010;152:726-732.

50. Moher D, Hopewell S, Schulz KF, et al. CONSORT 2010 Explanation and elaboration: updated guidelines for reporting parallel group randomised trials. *BMJ.* 2010;340:c869.

51. Chan A-W, Tetzlaff JM, Altman DG. SPIRIT 2013 statement: defining standard protocol items for clinical trials. *Ann Intern Med.* 2013;158(3):200-207.

52. Chan W, Tetzlaff JM, Gøtzsche PC, et al. SPIRIT 2013 explanation and elaboration: guidance for protocols of clinical trials. *BMJ.* 2013;346:e7586.

53. von Elm E, Altman DG, Egger M, et al. The Strengthening the Reporting of Observational Studies in Epidemiology (STROBE) statement: guidelines for reporting observational studies. *PLoS Med.* 2007;4(10):e296.

54. Vandenbroucke JP, von Elm E, Altman DG, et al. Strengthening the Reporting of Observational Studies in Epidemiology (STROBE): explanation and elaboration. *PLoS Med.* 2007;4(10):e297.

55. Stroup DF, Berlin JA, Morton SC, et al. Meta-analysis of observational studies in epidemiology: a proposal for reporting. *JAMA.* 2000;283(15):2008-2012.

56. Bossuyt PM, Reitsma JB, Bruns DE, et al. Towards complete and accurate reporting of studies of diagnostic accuracy: the STARD Initiative. *Radiology.* 2003;226:24-28.

57. Bossuyt PM, Reitsma, JB, Bruns DE, et al. STARD 2015: an updated list of essential items for reporting diagnostic accuracy studies. *BMJ.* 2015;351:h5527.

58. Cochrane A. *Effectiveness and Efficiency: Random Reflections on Health Services.* London: Nuffield Provincial Hospitals Trust; 1992.

59. Chalmers I. The Cochrane Collaboration: preparing, maintaining and disseminating systematic reviews of the effects of health care. *Ann NY Acad Sci.* 1993;703:156-163.

60. Grant MJ, Booth A. A typology of reviews: an analysis of 14 review types and associated methodologies. *Health Info Libr J.* 2009;26:91-108.

61. Liberati A, Altman DG, Tetzlaff J, et al. The PRISMA statement for reporting systematic reviews and meta-analyses of studies that evaluate healthcare interventions: explanation and elaboration. *BMJ.* 2009;339:b2700.

62. Thomas J, Harden A, Oakley A, et al. Integrating qualitative research with trials in systematic reviews. *BMJ.* 2004;328:1010-1012.

63. Booth A, Clarke M, Dooley G, et al. The nuts and bolts of PROSPERO: an international prospective register of systematic reviews. *Syst Rev.* 2012;1:2.
64. Moher D, Shamseer L, Clarke M, et al. Preferred reporting items for systematic review and meta-analysis protocols (PRISMA-P) 2015 statement. *Syst Rev.* 2015;4(1):1-8.
65. Moher D, Stewart L, Shekelle P. Establishing a new journal for systematic review products. *Syst Rev.* 2012;1:1-3.
66. Centers for Disease Control and Prevention. HIV and AIDS—United States, 1981–2000. http://www.cdc.gov/mmwr/pdf/wk/mm5021.pdf
67. Dukers NH, Goudsmit J, de Wit JB, Prins M, Weverling GJ, Coutinho RA. Sexual risk behaviour relates to the virological and immunological improvements during highly active antiretroviral therapy in HIV-1 infection. *AIDS.* 2001;15:369-378.
68. Arksey H, O'Malley L. Scoping studies: towards a methodological framework. *Int J Soc Res Methodol.* 2005;8(1):19-32.
69. Davis K, Drey N, Gould D. What are scoping studies? A review of the nursing literature. *Int J Nur Studies.* 2009;46(10):1386-1400.
70. Levac D, Colquhoun H, O'Brien KK. Scoping studies: advancing the methodology. *Implement Sci.* 2010;5:69-77.
71. Daudt, HM, Van Mossel, C, Scott, SJ. Enhancing the scoping study methodology: a large, inter-professional team's experience with the Arksey and O'Malley's framework. *BMC Med Res Methodol.* 2013;13:48-56.
72. Pham MT, Rajić A, Greig JD, Sargeant JM, Papadopoulos A, McEwen SA. A scoping review of scoping reviews: advancing the approach and enhancing the consistency. *Res Synth Methods.* 2014;5(4):371-385.
73. Shojania KG, Sampson M, Ansari MT, Ji J, Doucette S, Moher D. How quickly do systematic reviews go out of date? A survival analysis. *Ann Intern Med.* 2007;147:224-233.
74. Elliott JH, Turner T, Clavisi O, et al. Living systematic reviews: an emerging opportunity to narrow the evidence-practice gap. *PLoS Med.* 2014;11(2):e1001603.
75. Cochrane Community Archive. *Glossary: Cochrane Handbook for Systematic Reviews of Interventions 4.2.5.* http://www.cochrane.org/resources/glossary.htm. Updated May 2005.

CHAPTER 2

Basic Concepts

This chapter has three goals: (1) to discuss the basic concepts in a review of the literature, (2) to describe the structure of a typical research paper published in a health sciences journal in order to show where information can be found, and (3) to demonstrate how to conduct a methodological review of source documents using the Methods Map. At the end of this chapter, there are exercises to help you (a) determine what you need to know and where that information can be found in a peer-reviewed paper in a health sciences journal, and (b) apply what you have learned in carrying out a methodological review of a scientific paper.

This chapter consists of the following sections:

- Source Materials Defined
- Different Kinds of Source Materials
- Anatomy of a Scientific Paper: Finding What You Need in a Typical Research Paper
- A Methodological Review of the Literature: The Methods Map
- Caroline's Quest: Learning the Concepts
- What You Should Know or Be Able to Do by the End of This Chapter

SOURCE MATERIALS DEFINED

Source materials are publications and other documents about scientific knowledge that are analyzed in a review of the literature. Examples include papers published in scientific journals, reference books, or chapters in books, textbooks, and reports published by governmental and nongovernmental agencies and organizations.

DIFFERENT KINDS OF SOURCE MATERIALS

Primary, Secondary, and Tertiary Source Materials

An understanding of the differences between primary, secondary, and tertiary source materials is important in selecting documents for a literature review.

Primary Source Materials

Primary source materials are original research papers written by the scientists who conducted the study. An example of primary source material is the description of the purpose, methods, and results sections of a research paper in a scientific journal by the authors who designed and carried out the study.

A review of the scientific literature is based on the assumption that primary source materials have been examined and analyzed. You handicap yourself if you do not use primary source materials because the details of a study may be missing or misinterpreted in a summary about the study. Alternatively, secondary and tertiary source materials might prove to be very useful in the search for relevant primary source materials.

Secondary Source Materials

Secondary source materials are papers or other documents that summarize the original work of others. In other words, secondary source materials are based on information from primary source materials. Although secondary source materials are often written by individuals other than those who actually did the research, it is possible for authors to summarize their own previously published papers and those summaries are usually considered secondary source materials.

Examples of secondary source materials include a summary of previously published research in the introduction of a scientific research paper published in a journal, a description of what is known about a disease or treatment in a chapter in a reference book, or a synthesis based on a review of the literature.

Tertiary Source Materials

Tertiary source materials consist of a systematic analysis, meta-analysis, or critical review of scientific papers. The boundaries between secondary and tertiary source materials are not hard and fast; rather, they merge from one into another and differ in the degree of critical analysis as the review moves from secondary to tertiary. The term itself has not been standardized.

The availability of tertiary source materials has evolved over the past 25 years. With the veritable explosion of scientific knowledge and the rapid rise in the number of new sources, scientists and practitioners alike have been forced to not only stay abreast of new information but also to find more efficient ways to abstract, synthesize, and critically evaluate that knowledge. Tertiary source materials provide a variety of ways to accomplish the task of qualitative and quantitative evaluation of research findings.

Often tertiary source materials have a specific focus. Examples include papers or articles, like a critical review of all randomized clinical trials on a specific subject (such as the those in a Cochrane Review), a meta-analysis, practice guidelines, or papers that support evidence-based medicine on a clinical topic.

Publications

Traditionally source materials have been published in books or scientific journals that assume a permanence of documentation and are usually publicly accessible through libraries. This format has changed in recent years to include journals published in an electronic format on the Internet. For example, Internet resources include primary source papers in peer-reviewed scientific journals and secondary source documents such as those in annual reviews. This is true for qualitative as well as quantitative studies. Regardless of how the results of a scientific study are communicated, a basic requirement of source materials is public accessibility.

Not all materials that are publicly accessible are free. There may be a charge, depending on the source. Or source documents may not be available to the public at all. Examples include proprietary materials (those owned by individuals or organizations for their exclusive use), secret documents (such as those marked "classified" by the government), or confidential reports that cannot be accessed by people outside of a company or without a security clearance. Generally, documents such as these are not used as source materials in published, peer-reviewed journals. In other words, if you have access to such materials but those who read your review do not, then those restricted materials probably should not be included in a review of the literature.

Peer Review

Modern scientific inquiry carries the twofold assumption that progress is built on previous knowledge, and the methods and results of research are documented and available for all to inspect and study. A basic expectation of a paper describing original research, especially in scientific journals, is that it has been evaluated through the peer-review process. A peer is a person with the same (or superior) expertise in a scientific subject as the authors of the research article. A peer-reviewed paper, whether a primary, secondary, or tertiary publication, is one that has undergone the scrutiny of one or more scientific experts. Although peer review provides one kind of quality control in the scientific process, it is not the only measure of scientific quality, nor is it a guarantee of excellence. People who read the scientific literature must decide for themselves whether each study meets the standards of the research community.

The usual source for determining if a journal is peer reviewed is to consult Ulrich's International Periodical Directory (available in both print and electronic forms). If Ulrich's is not available or hard to use online, here are some other ways of finding out if a journal is peer reviewed:

1. Talk to a Reference Librarian. Although there is an online source for Ulrich's, sometimes it is difficult to access, even when you are searching within your own library. Unless you plan to use the printed version of Ulrich's at your library, the best way to find out if a journal is peer-reviewed is to call or make an appointment to meet with the reference librarian in a research library located in a university.

2. Go to Medline. Another possibility might be to assume that anything in Medline is usually peer reviewed, but not always. Check with the Reference Librarian.

3. Look at the Journal. You can also go online and check the masthead of a journal you are interested in. Do they have a board of editors, and are most of the editors based in universities? Then look to see if the journal says it is peer reviewed in its Instructions to Authors. If both of these conditions are met, then this is also probably a peer-reviewed journal.

Scientific Abstracts

A scientific abstract is an abbreviated summary of a study or theory. Abstracts of papers presented at scientific meetings are considered source materials, although they usually do not include enough information about the research methods to permit a reviewer to make a judgment about the scientific merit of the study. Presentations at scientific meetings can be primary source materials (if describing original research), secondary, or tertiary. Abstracts often are restricted in length and format—for example, no more than 250 to 500 words—and often are without citations of other research papers. For this reason some journals, such as the *Journal of the American Medical Association (JAMA)*, do not permit the inclusion of references to abstracts in a summary of a literature review in peer-reviewed journal articles. An example of an abstract presented at a professional meeting is shown in **Exhibit 2-1**.

> **EXHIBIT 2-1** Example of an Abstract in a Journal
>
> **Drug Use Management in Board and Care Facilities**
>
> *J. Garrard, S.L. Cooper, C. Goertz*
>
> Abstract: The purpose of this study was to describe medication management in board and care facilities throughout Minnesota. A triangulation of data collection methods was used, including mail questionnaires (N = 598 facilities), telephone interviews (N = 564 facilities), and site visits (N = 515 facilities). Major issues examined included characteristics of board and care facilities, staffing, residents, and drug management systems. Results showed that staff in 86% of the board and care facilities surveyed provided medication storage, 83% gave medication reminders, and 69% administered medications to one or more residents. Site visits revealed a wide diversity in the characteristics of managers and their attitudes toward medication administration.
>
> Data from Garrard J, Cooper SL, Goertz C. Drug use management in board and care facilities. *Gerontologist.* 1997; 37(6):748–756.[1]

For purposes of reviewing the literature, however, abstracts of papers from scientific meetings can be useful in several ways, such as the following:

- Alerting the reviewer to more recent scientific research, not yet published
- Providing useful leads to discovering other, more fully described studies in the peer-reviewed literature
- Identifying the name and location of researchers who can be contacted for further information

In many fields, abstracts of papers presented at scientific meetings are included in a special issue of the journal published by the society or organization that sponsored the meeting. Alternatively the abstracts may be issued in booklet form or electronically at the conference. In this case, the abstracts might be available to only those who attended the meeting. Contacting the author or someone who attended the meeting may be the only way of obtaining a copy of the abstracts. Recently some professional and scientific societies have begun to publish on the Internet a list of titles or abstracts of papers presented at national or international meetings. This possibility could be explored by searching the Internet for the website of the professional society and then determining whether the abstracts are available. A list of many professional societies and their websites is provided in Appendix A.

Citations, References, Bibliographies

A citation provides documentation about the source of an idea, statement, or research study referred to in a written document. Citations occur in the text or body of a scientific paper or book. A citation itself provides very little actual information; you have to go to the list of references or the bibliography (usually at the end of the paper or chapter in a book) to find out more about the document being cited.

Different formats for citations are used, depending on the preference of the journal or book. Two common formats are numerical and authors' last names. In the numerical format, the citation is given at the end of the cited material (or at the end of a sentence) as a superscript number. In the authors' last names format, the citation, usually located at the end of the sentence, is given as the last name of up to five authors, followed by et al., if more than five and the year of publication, enclosed in parentheses. These and other examples can be found in a style manual such as *Elements of Style*.[2] Examples of the numerical and authors' last names formats are shown in **Exhibit 2-2**.

A reference is the actual documentation of the work cited and should provide the information needed to find the work referred to. References are usually located at the end of a scientific paper or chapter in a book in the health sciences literature. See the end of this chapter for an example. The references of some documents, such as government reports or congressional records, are sometimes hard to decipher, and a reference librarian can be helpful in locating and understanding these materials.

Many different formats have been devised for the listing of references, and these differences have caused headaches for generations of students and researchers in the health sciences. Style manuals such as those by the American Psychological Association[3] (APA) and the American Medical Association[4] (AMA) can be used.

In writing your own papers, including a review of the literature, there are also computer software programs, such as EndNote, ProCite, or RefWorks, that

---

EXHIBIT 2-2 Examples of Formats of a Citation in a Research Paper

Numerical Format: These and other examples can be found in a style manual such as *The Elements of Style*.[26]

Authors' Last Names Format: These and other examples can be found in a style manual such as *The Elements of Style* (Strunk & White, 1979).

EXHIBIT 2-3 Examples of Formats for References

General Format

Authors. (Year of publication). Name of Book. City, State: Publisher.

Examples

Numerical Format:

26. Strunk W Jr, White EB. *The Elements of Style*. New York, NY: MacMillan; 1979.

Authors' Last Name Format:

Strunk, W., Jr., & White, E. B. (1979). *The elements of style*. New York, NY: MacMillan.

---

can be used to automatically convert a list of citations and lists of references into the correct format depending on which style you choose. Examples of two of the most common formatting styles used in listing references are shown in **Exhibit 2-3**. These two examples, numerical and authors' last name, correspond to the citations shown in Exhibit 2-2.

Several YouTube tutorials are available on the Internet, especially those by university libraries, which describe the APA style of citations and corresponding references. To find these, put the following in your browser: "YouTube citing scholarly articles using the APA style."

You can also search for variations of these instructions as written examples by going to the APA Style website and typing, "Learning APA Style." Also, at the APA Style homepage, scroll down to the bottom to Frequently Asked Questions about APA Style. In that section, under the term "References," there will be instructions for just about every imaginable type of reference you would possibly need. Check it out.

Alternatively, a non-YouTube tutorial on using the AMA style is located in the American Medical Association (AMA) Citation Style Guide. If you learn best by YouTube tutorials, then put the following in your search: "YouTube on how to cite scholarly articles using AMA style." Choose from among several by libraries or PubMed that have a YouTube tutorial. Formatting rules for citations and references to printed materials are fairly well known; however, similar rules for sources on the Internet have emerged only recently. Consult the style websites about how to cite sources on the Internet.

A bibliography, similar to a list of references, also includes references to books and other documents that are not quoted or cited in the text but are suggested for further reading. Authors often recommend additional materials for readers to consult if they want to develop a better understanding of the subject. Most scientific journals, however, do not encourage or allow bibliographies and limit the writers to lists of references cited in the text.

In summary, the distinctions between a citation, a reference, a list of references, and a bibliography can be described as follows:

- A **citation** is used in the body of a document to give credit to the publications of others or the author's own previous work.
- A **reference** for that citation gives complete information about how to find the materials, including the author(s) name, title of the scientific paper, the name and volume number of the journal, and the year of publication. A reference is usually located at the end of a scientific paper in health sciences journals.
- A **list of references** consists of all of the references that were cited in a scientific paper and is usually given at the end of a paper or book chapter. The references list may be numerical based on order in which the citation was cited (AMA style) or alphabetical by last name of the first author (APA) style. There are other variations about how the references are listed, depending on the scientific journal, or field, or other specifications.
- A **bibliography** consists of not only references, but also other books or papers that provide additional information about the subject being discussed. Most scientific journals restrict authors to references rather than bibliographies.

Hint

Whether writing a paper or a review of the literature, my first several drafts always use the APA style of citation because it is easier for me to find a particular reference in the alphabetical list of references at the end of the paper. Once I am further along in the draft, however, I switch to the AMA style of citation because it is more economical of space in the text (helps me to stay within the required number of pages) and is easier to find a particular reference in my References list at the end of the paper.

With the reference management software programs (e.g., End-Note, RefWorks), this switching back and forth between citation and their reference styles is very easy. This is my way of handling the issue; you may develop another based on your own experience.

With an understanding about how to cite the documents in your review of the literature based on either the APA or the AMA style, we now turn to two major topics of this chapter: (1) How to find what you need in a scientific paper and (2) how to determine the methodological qualifications of a study.

ANATOMY OF A SCIENTIFIC PAPER: FINDING WHAT YOU NEED IN A TYPICAL RESEARCH PAPER

Overview

Knowing where to find something is often as important as knowing what to do with it once you have found it. Research articles, especially those published in scientific journals, are the most common type of source materials used in reviews of the scientific literature. Most research articles follow a standard structure, which is described in this section. By knowing this structure, you will find it easier to locate different parts of the research study to abstract.

This is the first step in reviewing a scientific paper in a research journal, and eight sections in a scientific paper provide a framework for doing just that. In describing these eight sections, some additional comments have been included that might be useful to consider. These comments are set aside in boxes so they can easily be skipped by people with more experience in reading scientific literature.

Title and Authorship Section

The first section consists of the title of the paper and name and affiliations of the author or authors who conducted the research and wrote the paper. The affiliations of the authors are usually available in a special tab or at the end of the paper; this varies by journal.

The order of the authorship is important in most journals, with the first author usually being the person who had the most responsibility for the research paper. In some fields, the most senior scientist is listed last in order of authorship. This is often the person who provided the research mentorship, the laboratory, or the grant support for the research being reported; however, he or she may not have taken the primary responsibility for the paper being published. A third alternative is for the authors' names to be listed alphabetically. Knowledge of the field itself is needed to determine which protocol is followed in the peer-reviewed literature in health sciences journals.

Abstract Section

The abstract section consists of a brief summary of the paper which includes the purpose of the study, methods, results, and discussion. Although it is often identical in length and format to the abstract of a paper presented at a scientific meeting, the abstract section at the beginning of a scientific paper is just one part of the study described more fully in the remainder of the article. The abstract in a scientific paper is usually limited to 25 to 250 words.

Summarizing the abstract section of selected journal articles does *not* constitute a review of the literature because there are usually not enough details in this brief description to allow you to understand how the research was done or how to interpret the results.

Introduction Section

Generally the introduction section includes the following four major parts: (1) a brief summary of the authors' review of the literature; (2) the motivation for the paper (i.e., what is missing or unknown in the research literature up to the time the study began); (3) an overview of the scientific theory or conceptual models on which the research was based; and (4) the purpose of the research study described in the paper. Depending on the journal or the author, the purpose of a study can be in the form of a statement, a research question, or a hypothesis.

Sometimes authors seem to forget what their original purpose was (whether it was explicitly stated or not), especially in light of interesting results that may have answered another unstated research question. Alternatively authors may have satisfied the purpose they stated but then asked and answered additional research questions as the paper progresses. You have to decide for yourself whether the authors described a complete purpose in the introduction section of their paper and presented results about the purpose they stated in the introduction section.

Methods Section

The methods section is a description of the procedures used to carry out the research study and should be complete enough to permit another researcher to replicate the study without the need to contact the authors. The methods section of a typical scientific paper includes information about methodological design, subjects, data sources, data collection methods, and statistical and analytical procedures.

Methodological Design

This describes how the research was structured, including how a sample was formed, how many intervention or treatment groups there were, and, if more than one, how groups (experimental and control) were formed through the use of random assignment, self-selection, or some other strategy. This subsection should also include a description and definition of each of the major variables in the study, including the independent and dependent variables and the covariates. Some studies will not have an independent variable or a covariate, but all have one or more dependent variables.

Subjects

This is a description of how the subjects were chosen for the study—the inclusion and exclusion criteria, sampling design, number of subjects included in the study and their characteristics, such as gender, age, and disease status. This subsection may also include a description of how many individuals were initially selected; the number who actually participated in the study; and differences between those chosen, those who agreed to participate, those who dropped out, and those who participated at each stage of the research. Be forewarned, however, many older studies do not report this level of detail about the attrition rates among subjects. Instead, they simply report the number of subjects in the final statistical analyses. Increasingly, this lack of information about subjects from point of recruitment to final analysis is considered a lack of scientific rigor, given the standards that have been published since the early 2000s.

Data Sources

This subsection is an explanation of whether the information about the subjects in the study was based on primary source data, secondary source data, or both. Primary source data are gathered by the researchers who are reporting the study; secondary source data were usually gathered by others.

Primary and secondary source data should not be confused with primary and secondary source materials as described at the beginning of this chapter. If secondary source data are used, then the authors should include a description of the characteristics of the database; the original reason the data were gathered (e.g., as administrative records or as claims files for health care reimbursement); and the dates during which the data were gathered. Some studies include both primary and secondary source data. For example, primary source data might be information from a survey of the subjects by the researchers, which the same researchers then combined with secondary source data, such as clinical records obtained from the medical charts that were recorded by the treating physicians, and use of data from both sources can be an excellent methodological strategy.

Data Collection Methods

This is a description of all of the data collection instruments used in primary source data collection. In this subsection of a journal article, the questionnaire, survey, interview protocol, or other data collection instrument is described, including either the results of validity and reliability analyses of the data collection instrument itself or references to other studies that include such information.

Statistical and Analytical Procedures

This subsection describes the types of statistical tests or analytical procedures used and the assumptions underlying their use, if applicable.

Not all research papers published in health-related journals include these five subsections in a methods section, and even if they are included, they may not be in the order described here. Also, a method that is not described in the methods section may be mentioned later in the results section.

The choice and order of subsections in the methods section of a scientific paper depend on the field, the content, the type of study, and choices made by the individual author.

The appearance of a previously unannounced set of methods in the results or discussion section may suggest a lack of tidiness in the authors' style of reporting. Alternatively such a practice may be entirely appropriate if the results of the main research question suggested to the researchers that they should explore something further and the methods for that exploration are then described.

Results Section

The results section presents the results of the study, and in so doing, answers the research question, verifies or refutes the hypothesis, or addresses the purposes of the study that should have been stated in the introduction section. This may be the shortest section of the entire paper, and the details may be presented concisely in one or more tables or figures.

The results section may require the most intensive reading in order to understand the findings fully. Some journals limit this section only to results; others allow authors to discuss their interpretation of the findings in this section. If interpretations are included, you must be sure to distinguish the actual results from the authors' interpretations or opinions.

Discussion and Conclusion Section

The discussion and conclusion section usually addresses these five areas:

1. Summary of the research study as it relates to the purpose or research question or hypothesis originally described.
2. Interpretation and discussion of what these results mean. This is the part of the paper in which the authors can express their opinions about the interpretation of the findings.
3. Description of the strengths and weaknesses of the study, including methodological strengths and weaknesses.
4. Discussion of future research. Often the results of one study suggest additional research questions. A brief description of these topics may be included in this section of the paper.
5. Statement about the significance of this research study. This is not statistical significance but rather a description about the impact of the findings on clinical care or evidence-based practices.

As with other parts of a research paper, this discussion and conclusion section may not include all of these topics or be in the same order, and there may also be other topics not included in this discussion.

List of References

The list of references is a listing of all of the papers or other sources cited by the authors in describing previous or related research. This list is very important in adding new papers to your own review of the literature. Read the References section carefully to see if other papers in your area of interest are present and look them up yourself.

Acknowledgments Section

This section includes a description of how the research study was funded, for example, the names of granting agencies or foundations and the names of individuals who assisted in the research or review. If the research was funded by the National Institute of Health (NIH), then the paper should be available in the PubMed Central (NIH) database.

These eight sections are usually found in most journal articles in peer-reviewed literature and constitute, what I call, the anatomy of a scientific article. But what do you know about the study itself? How can you judge whether this study was good or not? Isn't that the essence of a critical review?

Yes, it definitely is, and you need courses in research methods and statistics to make such judgments. But which comes first in your learning process: methods courses and then how to review the literature, or the other way around? I shall assume that it is the other way around. You will get to those important courses (if you haven't already). In the meantime, you still need an outline of the essential steps about the design and implementation of a research study to evaluate that study in a literature review. This is the topic of the next section in this chapter.

A METHODOLOGICAL REVIEW OF THE LITERATURE: THE METHODS MAP

Overview

Once you know the structure of a scientific paper and how to find what you need, the second step is understanding what research methods the authors used to carry out their study. In this section, I describe some fundamentals about research methodologies used in many of the health-related journals. A review of the literature can be done from a number of different perspectives, such as variations in the theories on which the studies were based, the hypotheses tested, or a comparison of research results. But underlying all of these perspectives is a description of the research methodology, which is the framework for most empirical studies. A list of potential topics for examining the empirical literature is provided in **Exhibit 2-4**. To include all of these topics in your review of the

---

EXHIBIT 2-4 Methodological Topics for Reviewing Research Studies in the Health Sciences Literature

Purpose of the paper

Method

Research design
- Operational definition of variables
- Independent and dependent variables
- Intervention
- Methodological design
- Random assignment

Data collection instruments and procedures
- Data sources
- Data collection designs
  - Pre-post design
  - Prospective/retrospective
  - Longitudinal/cross-sectional
- Data collection instruments
  - Author-designed instruments
  - Standardized instruments
  - Other instrument
- Instrument characteristics (number of items, format)
- Psychometric characteristics of data collection instruments
  - Validity studies about the instrument
  - Reliability studies about the instrument
- Setting

Subjects
- Unit of analysis
- Selection criteria, including inclusion and exclusion criteria
- Random selection of subjects
- Sampling design
- Subject characteristics
- Number of subjects (in description or by flowchart)
  - Participation and attrition rates
  - Participant/nonparticipant differences

Data analysis
- Statistical methods
- Statistical assumptions

Results

Discussion/conclusion
- Interpretation of results
- Strengths and weaknesses
- Significance of results (practical or clinical)
- Conclusions

References

Acknowledgments

literature might be excessive, but you can use this list to decide which topics you want to emphasize in your review.

In order to understand what the topics in Exhibit 2-4 mean, the Methods Map is introduced here and used throughout the remainder of this chapter.

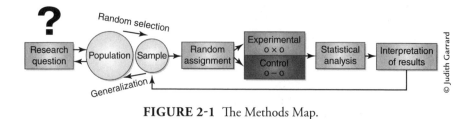

FIGURE 2-1 The Methods Map.

The Methods Map describes some of the major decisions that researchers need to make about the design of a research study in the health sciences. An understanding of these methodological decisions will not only help you analyze what the authors did but also what they did not do.

Figure 2-1 is the Methods Map. I created this map to help students visualize the process of designing and implementing a research study. This schematic shows each of the major stages of a study and some of the methodological choices that need to made. The map itself can change depending on what the researchers actually did. For example, they may not have used random assignment of subjects to groups; in that case, the reader can change the label to "self-assignment by subjects" on the map. Alternatively the researchers may have studied only one group of subjects, thus there would be only one group rather than two groups (experimental and control) on the map.

In reviewing the literature, the Methods Map serves as a useful checklist to see how authors handled these methodological decisions. As used throughout this chapter, each part of the map is highlighted as I explain what those decisions were. I will begin with a brief description of the *process* of designing a research study, using different points of interest on the Methods Map, and continue afterward with a description of major decisions about each of these stages.

The Process of a Research Study

In the following thumbnail sketch of the process, follow the Methods Map in Figure 2-1 using the **words in bold**.

Begin at the left of the map with the **research question** of the study. Next, think about the **population** of subjects to whom this question will apply.

If researchers have access to the population, then they may use **random selection** from the population to create a **sample** for this study. If random selection is not possible, they need to obtain as representative a sample of the population as possible.

The **sample** of subjects includes a description of the unit of analysis, criteria for inclusion and exclusion of eligible subjects, number of subjects, and their characteristics (e.g., age, gender, race or ethnicity). Next, determine how many groups of subjects the sample will be assigned to. If there are two or more groups (perhaps **experimental** and **control**), then how will subjects be assigned to those groups? **Random assignment** of subjects to groups is the gold standard in the health sciences literature. The **experimental group** gets the intervention of interest (symbolized by an **X**) and the **control group** (symbolized by a dash, –) gets something else or a placebo. There can be one, two, or many groups (consisting of multiple experimental and control groups), with different kinds of intervention, depending on the research question.

The layout of the groups of subjects (**experimental** and **control**) also symbolizes **when the data were collected** with the use of an **O (for observation)**. Data collection is an important part of any study and encompasses at least three major questions: (1) what data collection instrument was used, (2) what were its psychometric characteristics, and (3) when were the data collected? The Methods Map shows two data collection points for each group: pretest (before the intervention—placebo) and posttest (after the intervention—placebo). When all of the posttest data have been collected, **statistical analysis** is conducted to analyze the findings.

Interpretation of results, which includes both the statistical results and the impact on the subjects, is the final stage in which authors provide their explanation about what the results mean for each research question. This interpretation of results is usually in the discussion section of the paper.

The **arrow** on the Methods Map, from the **interpretation of results** back to the original **sample** of subjects, shows to whom the results and interpretations apply. Thus initially, the results and interpretation of the study are **applicable to the sample** (that is, all subjects in the sample) and then back through the chain to the **population** (but only if **random selection** of the sample was used). Application of results to the population is known as **generalization** to the population. From there, researchers use the results and interpretations to answer the **research question** they began with. If random selection was not used, then the results of the statistical analysis and interpretation are applied only to the **sample**. Finally, it is common knowledge in the scientific community that a study is not completed until it is published in the peer-reviewed literature, and those peer-reviewed papers are what you examine in your review of the literature.

Does the process of designing a study really work that way? Not exactly. The design and implementation of a research study rarely follow in such a linear or step-by-step fashion. For example, researchers often return to the initial research question throughout the study—refining, limiting, or restating it as they think through each of the subsequent steps. What you see in the published paper is a final statement of the research question, not all the revisions or even the original question. Sometimes researchers cannot randomly assign subjects to groups or even create two or more groups of subjects. As you review each paper, consider the possibility that every choice, every step, everything done requires a decision by the researchers. Identifying and dealing with those problems are the topics of many methods courses. That knowledge plus experience and the best possible solutions under practical circumstances become the art of conducting research. In general, the Methods Map outlines some of the major issues the researcher needs to consider. Next, I will concentrate on each part of the Methods Map in greater detail.

What Is the Purpose of the Study?

In describing a research study, researchers should begin with **the purpose of the study** or **research question**, as shown in **Figure 2-2**. As the study proceeds, researchers will return to this question repeatedly. This question guides the way in which the study is thought about and how the design is laid out.

As you review the literature, state this purpose in question form in your own words and decide whether the question actually changed as you review the paper.

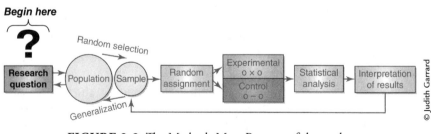
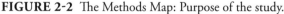

FIGURE 2-2 The Methods Map: Purpose of the study.

Why did the authors do this particular study? What was their purpose or hypothesis or research question? Distinguish between what they said (or implied) their purpose was in the introduction section of the paper and what they actually addressed or answered in the results section.

> The authors may describe the purpose in the form of a general statement, a hypothesis, or a research question. A mark of poor research quality is a paper that does not specifically state the purpose of the study in the introduction section.

What Is the Population?

After the research question is known, it is important think about the **population** of subjects the question should apply to. If access to the population is possible, then researchers can select from the population the individuals who will actually be the subjects in the sample. The decisions about how to select subjects made at this point are crucial. Ideally most researchers would like to use **random selection** to choose which subjects will be in the **sample**. That ideal situation is shown in **Figure 2-3**. But often it is not possible to randomly select subjects from a population.

If random sampling was not used to create the sample of subjects at the beginning of the study, it is theoretically not possible to generalize the results back to the population after the study is completed. Think of this as a two-way bridge: if researchers have not gone over the bridge one way (from the population to the sample) at the beginning of the study, they cannot go back over the bridge at the end of the study to generalize the results of the study to the population (from the sample to the population).

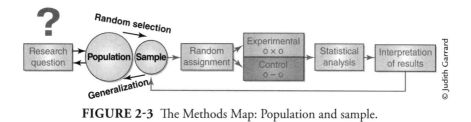

FIGURE 2-3 The Methods Map: Population and sample.

The theoretical underpinnings that allow researchers to randomly sample from the population to generate a representative sample are based on probability theory, as described in statistics textbooks; the topic is beyond the scope of this text. By the same token, generalization from the sample to the population is based on assumptions about statistical methods. Again, it is well beyond this chapter, but the theory is there. The bottom line is this: if researchers have not generated a random sample, they are theoretically prohibited from generalizing the results of the study to the population.

Whether the sample has been randomly selected from the population or not, researchers *must* have a sample of subjects to proceed with the study. As you review each paper, read it carefully to determine for yourself if a random sample was generated. Do not assume that the sample is a random sample if the authors did not describe the steps they went through to generate such a sample from the population.

Who Are the Subjects in the Sample?

The **sample** in **Figure 2-4** represents a number of decisions by the researchers, including at the very least these four: the unit of analysis, inclusion and exclusion criteria for defining an eligible subject, number of subjects, and subject characteristics.

Unit of Analysis

As you review the literature, first determine who or what the unit of analysis was in the study. Examples of the different units of analysis are the following:

- Individual: The subject of the study is an individual being. Because most studies are of humans, this would be an individual person. For example, in a study

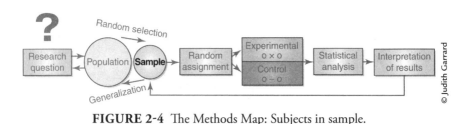

FIGURE 2-4 The Methods Map: Subjects in sample.

of smoking behavior of children, a child would be the unit of analysis. Thus the number of subjects would be the number of individuals in the sample.

- Group: The subject is a group of people. For example, in a study of the relationship between family size and group cohesiveness, the family would be the unit of analysis. Thus the number of subjects would be the number of families in the sample.
- Organization: The subject is an organization, such as a health department or school or hospital. For example, a study of state health departments throughout the United States that do or do not have prevention programs for HIV/AIDS would use the health department as the unit of analysis. Thus the number of subjects would be the number of health departments in the sample.
- Social artifact: A social artifact has been defined in the research literature as the product of a social being. Examples of social artifacts include a health care policy or law or a practice guideline, something different from the other three units of analysis. An example of research in which a social artifact is the subject would be a study of the characteristics of state guidelines on vaccination of preschool children. The state guideline (which is a social artifact) would be the unit of analysis for this study. Thus the number of subjects would be the number of state guidelines in the sample (assuming each state had only one official guideline).

> Most, but not all, studies in the health and behavioral sciences use an individual as the unit of analysis. If another unit of analysis was used, it is important to determine how the researchers operationally defined that unit. For example, if an organization, such as a hospital, was the unit of analysis, did the researchers define what they meant by a hospital in terms such as bed size, geographic area, or type of ownership? In this example, record the role of the individual who spoke on behalf of the hospital, such as the chief financial officer or the medical director. But the spokesperson was not the unit of analysis; the hospital was.

Selection Criteria

As you review each study, determine what the rules of inclusion and exclusion were for selecting subjects for the study. The researchers should provide that information. If not, try to define the criteria as you read the study.

An example of inclusion criteria is age range and type of health plan: only people between the ages of 18 and 64 years who were enrolled in a managed health care organization qualified for the study. Thus the exclusion criteria would be people whose ages were less than 18 years or greater than 64 years and those who had some other kind of health care plan or no health care plan at all.

Number of Subjects

As you review the literature, try to account for all subjects in the original sample. Researchers should not decrease the sample size just because subjects wandered off, died, refused to come to any more sessions, or did not respond to the invitation to be in the sample. Make sure that you can account for *everybody* in the sample. The number of subjects in a study is often abbreviated as $(N = x)$, where x is the number. For example, in a study with five subjects, they might use $(N = 5)$ in the statistical analysis tables.

Summarizing the number of subjects can involve other related questions that may be important to your review of the literature. Here are a few:

- Participation and attrition rates: What was the total number of subjects the researchers began with compared to the number who left during the study and the final number of subjects who completed the study? These enumerations can be surprisingly difficult to find in a scientific paper.

The original number of subjects is a fundamental piece of information that some authors fail to provide; therefore, you might consider noting the total number or its absence in every study in your review. If there is more than one group of subjects, for example, an experimental (E) group and a control (C) group, then record the number of subjects in each group in this cell of your matrix, for example: E $(N = 126)$, C $(N = 140)$.

- Participant and nonparticipant differences: What information was given about the differences between people who stayed in the study and those who either refused to be in the study in the first place or left before the study ended?

A similar discussion about participant and nonparticipant differences might be in terms of the dropout rate or respondent and nonrespondent analysis.

- Absence of information: Equally noteworthy is the absence of a description of such differences. This is an important issue that concerns the possibility of bias in the final group of subjects for whom data were analyzed.

Subject Characteristics

Which subject characteristics did the authors describe? Examples include gender, age range, race or ethnicity, or other characteristics such as disease status, geographic location, or socioeconomic status.

> In generating a sample, researchers are usually looking forward in time, getting ready to create experimental and control groups. As you review the literature, however, it is important to know the characteristics of the subjects at both the beginning and the end of the study. Were the characteristics of the subjects at the beginning the same as the characteristics of those who completed the study? The researchers may not have described this, but in your review of the literature you should note the differences (if the information is available in the paper).

What Is the Methodological Design of the Study?

In **Figure 2-5**, a methodological design is shown in which there are two groups of subjects; one is the **experimental group**, the other is the **control group**. These groups were formed by **random assignment** of subjects from the original sample. As shown in the Methods Map, **point A** covers both random assignment and these two groups. This design is not the only possibility, however.

In reviewing the literature, you need to determine which design was used in the study. The design can change within a paper, depending on which research

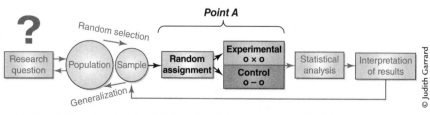

FIGURE 2-5 The Methods Map: Random assignment of subjects to groups.

question was being asked, and there can also be several research questions, each with its own design, in any one study.

Random Assignment of Subjects to Groups

Ideally researchers **randomly assign** all the subjects in the sample to either the experimental group or the control group. If there is only one group (presumably the only group that received the intervention, with no control group), then all the subjects in the sample would be assigned to that one group. In some designs there may be two or more groups, and subjects chose which group to go to. In that case there is no random assignment of subjects to groups.

There are some other rules about subjects and groups. No subject can be assigned to more than one group, and after a subject is assigned to a group, the subject is supposed to stay in that group (not switch from the control group to the experimental group, for example). The issue here is *how* the subjects get into those groups—either by random assignment or nonrandom assignment (subjects or someone else chooses which one they go to, but not by random assignment). This, too, is a crucial decision point.

The Methods Map shows an ideal situation (**random assignment** to **experimental** and **control** groups), but that may not be the case for the study you are reviewing. Substitute here whatever design was used, including whether or not subjects were randomly assigned to groups.

> Technically the term *experimental design* implies random assignment of subjects to groups, but recent usage has become a bit lax. Ask yourself whether the authors specifically said the subjects were randomized, or randomly assigned, if they said they used an experimental design. A general rule is: if the authors knew enough about methodological designs to randomly assign subjects to groups, then they should have known enough to describe how they did it in the methodology section.

Methodological Designs

The following methodological designs are commonly used in the behavioral sciences. They are in descending order of their ability to detect a difference between two or more groups of subjects:

- Experimental designs: These designs are characterized by random assignment of subjects to two or more groups (an experimental group and a control group). This is the strongest design for detecting a difference between the groups.

- Quasi-experimental designs: Quasi means *almost*, as in *almost an experimental design*. These designs do not include random assignment of subjects to groups and thus are less rigorous than experimental designs.
- Pre-experimental designs: Pre-experimental designs not only lack random assignment of subjects to groups but also have methodological problems that limit researchers from some of the conclusions that can be made about the results.
- Observational designs: Although these are useful designs, they do not have the methodological power of even the pre-experimental designs because they usually include only one group of subjects. But observational designs are an important first step in carefully examining a research question. You will see these are used most often when a new topic of scientific interest is first described. The forte of this design is the specific definition and description of the problem, such as the initial studies of patients' symptoms to a newly emerging antibiotic-resistant disease.

The behavioral sciences use these four major designs in empirical studies: experimental, quasi-experimental, pre-experimental, and observational. In epidemiological studies, other designs are used or are described in different terms, including randomized controlled trials, case-control designs, cohort designs, and cross-sectional designs. Qualitative designs, such as those that use focus groups, are another kind of design.[5] See the texts by Campbell and Stanley[6] and Cook and Campbell[7] for a description of behavioral sciences designs. Kleinbaum, Kupper, and Morgenstern[8] describe the epidemiological designs.

How Do Random Selection and Random Assignment Differ?

Random assignment is what differentiates experimental designs from designs in the other categories in both the behavioral sciences and in epidemiology. The purpose of random assignment is to create two or more subject groups that are as equal as possible at the beginning of an experimental study, that is, before an intervention is applied. Usually one of these groups is designated as the experimental group; the other is the control group. Random assignment is a methodological design issue.

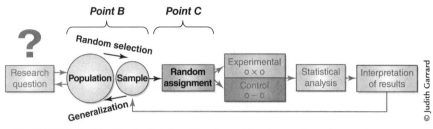

FIGURE 2-6 The Methods Map: Random selection and random assignment.

Random selection is concerned with the selection of a representative sample of subjects from a population. Random selection is a sampling design issue. Sometimes there is confusion between random selection and random assignment. The Methods Map will help in this explanation.

Random selection occurs when a sample of subjects is selected from the population of subjects. That is at **point B** in **Figure 2-6**.

Random assignment of subjects to groups occurs when the researchers decide what to do with that sample of subjects (once they have them) by distributing them (randomly) to two or more groups in a methodological design. Random assignment of subjects to groups is shown at **point C** in Figure 2-6.

The word *random* occurs in both **random selection** and **random assignment**. Random is the best research tool available for avoiding bias in both cases. But random selection and random assignment are two distinct acts at different points in the design of a study. The best way to keep them separate is to use these terms as you review a paper:

- Random **selection of subjects from the population to create the sample**—remember to say the bold part. In random selection, you are going from the population to the sample. You begin with the population:
  Population → Sample
- Random **assignment of subjects to two or more groups in the methodological design**—here you are starting with the sample and going from it to two or more groups. You begin with the sample already selected:
  Sample → Groups (experimental and control groups)

They differ in what you start with (either the population or the sample) and where you are going (either to the sample or the groups). The sample you begin with does not need to have been randomly selected in order for you to randomly assign subjects to two or more groups. That is why many studies do not have a random sample but they do use random assignment to create two or more (theoretically) equal groups. Saying that a study was a randomized controlled trial (RCT) says only that once you have a sample (either with or without random sampling), then you used random assignment in that study to assign subjects to groups. Again, you do not have to have randomly selected the sample in order create an RCT. But the authors should be very careful about how that sample was created in the first place.

What Are the Independent and Dependent Variables?

A general definition of a variable is a concrete representation of an abstraction. In other words, a variable is the name for something, whether it exists in physical form or not. We might have something concrete, like my office chair or your dining room chair, or we can have the *concept* of a chair. If this concept includes two or more attributes, then it is a variable. Thus, we could define *chair* as consisting of many different kinds of chairs—office chair, kitchen chair, living room chair, high chair, and so forth. The general concept is the variable. The variations are the attributes of that variable.

In reviewing the literature, it is important to understand how the two specific kinds of variables, independent and dependent variables, enable us to analyze what methodological design was used. Here is how they are defined:

- Independent variable: The independent variable is the one that researchers have control over. That means they can assign one group of subjects to get an intervention and other group to get the placebo or nonintervention.
- There may or may not be an independent variable in a study. If there is only one group of subjects, then there is no independent variable because there are no variations in the groups. In other words, there were no attributes. Alternatively, a single study may have multiple independent variables.
- Dependent variable: The dependent variable measures the outcomes or the results of the study.
- A study will always have a dependent variable. In reviewing the literature, you first need to ask yourself, What is the dependent variable? There can be multiple dependent variables in a study.

Let's pause a minute and look at what I am calling *an intervention*. It could be the condition assigned to the experimental group and not to the control group, or it could be what a single group got in a one-group study.

An example of an intervention in a study of a diabetes education program could be the program presented to the experimental subjects; another program was presented to the control group. The dependent variable in such a study could be a measure of the subject's diabetes condition, such as the value of an HbA1c for each subject at the end of the study. Better yet, the dependent variable could be done on a pre-post-test basis (before and after the study) and the measure could be the difference between the pretest and the posttest values.

Sometimes interventions are not applied by the researchers themselves. The intervention may be some external event, such as a change in health policy or a drug formulary change, and the purpose of the study is to examine the effects of such a change.

An intervention might be a Medicare regulation, such as a restriction on the use of specific medications in nursing homes. In this example the experimental group consisted of the nursing homes under the federal regulation that got the intervention, and the comparison group comprised homes that were not under the regulation and got the usual care or some other program. In these kinds of studies, the author is expected to give a clear description of the externally applied intervention. Sometimes such a description is not given because it is so well known in the field; if this is the case, there should be at least a reference to a book or journal article, or other document or source material, that describes the well-known intervention. Finally, some studies may have only one group of subjects, all of whom experienced the same intervention. In that case, there is no independent variable, although there should definitely be a dependent variable.

Let's use the Methods Map to better understand how independent and dependent variables can be represented in a methodological design.

As shown in **Figure 2-7**, the arrow for the **independent variable** shows two attributes: **X** and – (dash). These two attributes (X and –) represent the differences

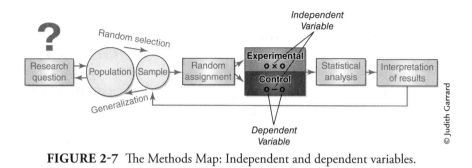

FIGURE 2-7 The Methods Map: Independent and dependent variables.

in intervention between the experimental group and the control group. In other words, each of those groups represents a different attribute of the independent variable. If there was only one group in the study, then that group would get the intervention, but there would be no independent variable.

As you review a study, lay out subject groups in the methodological design. How many groups were there? Did each group differ from the others in the treatment or intervention they received? Perhaps one group received the program of interest (the experimental group), the second group received a different kind of treatment (control group 1), and the third group received usual care (control group 2). In this case, there was an independent variable (type of treatment) with three attributes (experimental treatment, another treatment, and usual care).

In deciding whether there was an independent variable in a study, look to see how many groups of subjects there were for each research question. Two or more groups is often (but not always) an indication that there was an independent variable, and the different ways the groups were treated were likely to be the attributes of that variable.

The bottom line is that a variable has to vary, that is, it has to have two or more attributes. Look to see how many groups of subjects there are and how they differed, and use that as a clue to identifying the attributes of an independent variable.

The arrow for the **dependent variable** points to the **O**s (for observation of data). This includes all of the Os, that is, all of the observations or testing of subjects in the study. In Figure 2-7, the researchers had four observations (Os) of the dependent variable: two for the experimental group (pre- and posttests) and two for the control group (pre- and posttests). The Os show *when* the dependent variable was measured. The attributes of the dependent variable are how the subjects varied on the variable itself.

Here is an example. The purpose of a study was to determine which of two types of surgical procedures resulted in the least amount of pain as measured in the outcome variable (the dependent variable). One group of subjects received procedure A (the experimental group), and the other group received procedure B (the control group). The outcome measure was a pain scale that patients used to rate their pain on a scale of 0 to 10. Each of the subjects in both groups was asked to rate his or her pain at that point in time from 0 (no pain) to 10 (the worst pain they ever experienced) before and after the surgical procedures. Thus, the researchers looked at the differences between pre- and posttesting to compare procedures A and B.

The independent variable in this study was type of surgical procedure (A or B), and the dependent variable was the pain scale. The attributes of the independent variable (what distinguished the experimental group from the control group) was type of surgical procedure (A or B). The attributes of the dependent variable were the different ratings (0 to 10) on the pain scale. The Os of the dependent variable in the Methods Map show when the pain scale was administered (pretest and posttest).

When and How Will Data Be Collected?

In **Figure 2-8** we are at the point labeled **data collection**. What the map shows is *when* the data were collected (pre- and posttesting) in a methodological design consisting of two groups (experimental and control) differentiated by the attributes of the independent variable (X and –).

What is *not* shown in the Methods Map are the details about the data collection instrument itself and how it was used in this study. That information

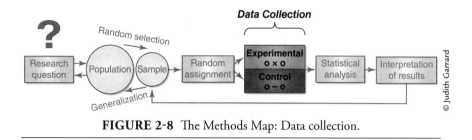

FIGURE 2-8 The Methods Map: Data collection.

is an important part of your review and can usually be found in the methods section of the paper. In your review of the literature you can analyze differences between studies on the basis of one or more data collection instruments, discussed next.

Data Collection Instruments and Procedures

Your first question about data collection should be about the data collection instrument itself. Examples include questionnaires, surveys, and administrative or clinical records. Other kinds of data collection methods are focus groups,[5] the Delphi technique, or an interview protocol that the researchers developed (which they should describe in detail).

In the language of data collection, an instrument can be a questionnaire or a list of interview questions, sometimes called a *protocol*, or a set of instructions for recording certain behaviors about subjects by the person observing those subjects. For example, a questionnaire might consist of questions about different kinds of foods, and subjects are asked to check off each food they use. An interview protocol is generally a set of questions that the researcher asks of each subject. The wording and the order of the questions are both important, and the interviewer usually is not allowed to deviate from that order or provide spontaneous supplemental information to the subjects. Some basic reference books that might be useful include those on questionnaire design,[9] conducting a survey,[10] and the design and use of focus groups.[5]

Data Sources

In addition to knowing about which data collection instrument was used, it is also important in a literature review to know if the data were primary or secondary. Primary source data consists of information gathered by the researchers (or their research assistants) who conducted the original study; these are usually the authors of the paper you are reviewing. Alternatively, data gathered by other researchers or for other purposes are called secondary source data.

Secondary source data can come in many forms. Some examples include information gathered for administrative purposes, such as data from patients upon admission to a hospital, records of reimbursement for health care services, or Medicare data about a health condition. If secondary source data were used, note in your review of the literature why the data were collected initially (health services claims files or as part of administrative records).

Another example of secondary source data gathered for purposes other than research includes information about a patient's symptoms gathered by clinicians in a medical center and recorded in an electronic clinical record. If a researcher used that information in a study of those patients, he or she would be using secondary source data. However, if the researcher surveys the patients directly about the same or a different set of symptoms, the data would be considered primary source data.

An example of a national secondary source data set is the National Health and Nutrition Examination Survey; see website: http://www .cdc.gov/nchs/nhanes.htm, which is a national survey about the health and nutritional status of Americans conducted by the National Center for Health Statistics. The initial survey was conducted in the early 1960s.

In some studies data from different sources are combined to create a database, and these data sources can be from primary or secondary sources, or both. For example, clinicians interested in the effects of a specific drug on the cognitive status of older patients may use a medical evaluation questionnaire they administered to gather primary source data from patients and then used data from the patients' insurance companies to gather additional information about health care costs. In this example, the two data sets, primary and secondary, would be linked through an individual identifier, such as the patient's name or code number.

Let me stop a minute here to again distinguish between primary/secondary source data (described in this section) and primary/secondary source papers (as described under Data Sources in the Anatomy of a Scientific Paper earlier in this chapter). The difference between source data and source papers is often raised by my own graduate students at this point in the discussion.

Primary source data are collected by the authors of the paper you are examining; **secondary source data** were gathered originally by someone else, either other researchers (which could have included the original authors) or an organization such as Medicare or by some other group of people (such as clinicians in another health care system). Secondary source data, such as results of clinical examinations, can be used and/or merged with primary source data in a database linked by some identifier, such as subjects' code numbers. Both primary and secondary source data are an important part of studies in the peer-reviewed literature.

Primary source documents are scientific papers or articles written by the authors who conducted the study. **Secondary source documents** are also scientific papers that are usually summarized by another group of scientists in a review of the literature or systematic review or meta-analysis or government report, etc. and described usually by that second set of authors (which may or may not include the original author). Both are important in the peer-reviewed literature.

Data Collection Designs

Record more details about when the data were collected, for example, "pre-post-post" for one pretesting and two posttestings, that is, one testing before the intervention and two testings after the intervention. Also determine whether the data were gathered prospectively or retrospectively. Were the data gathered at two or more points in time (possibly a longitudinal study) or at a single point in time (cross-sectional)?

Psychometric Characteristics of Data Collection Instruments

Record in your matrix whether results are reported about the validity and reliability of each data collection instrument. If the authors developed the instrument but no information was given about validity and reliability, then make a note of the lack of information about these fundamental psychometric characteristics.

Whether the data source is primary or secondary, or the data are quantitative or qualitative, or the measurement scale of each of the variables on the form is nominal, ordinal, interval, or ratio, the same question about the data collection instrument itself applies: Is there any documentation that the data collection *instrument* was valid and reliable?

Validity

Instrument validity asks: Are we measuring what we think we're measuring? Generally there are four kinds of instrument validity:

1. *Face validity*: Does the question look like it is asking what we mean to ask? This is the simplest level of instrument validity, but it can be a meaningful question. Sometimes we phrase this question by asking ourselves and others to look at each data collection item and ask: Is that what you mean? or Does the phrasing of that question or item make sense? Will it make sense to the subjects in the study?

   Sometimes we ask one question when we really want to ask another. For example, we might ask a patient, Are you satisfied with your life? when what we really want to know is, Are you feeling depressed? If an assessment of depression is what you intend, then a question about satisfaction with life probably lacks face validity.

2. *Content validity*: A second kind of instrument validity concerns the extent to which the items cover the issues on this topic. For example, health-related quality of life may have a number of facets, not all of which can be measured by just one or two questions. A data collection instrument may lack this kind of validity if it is too brief or fails to address the basics of an issue or topic. Content validity was initially discussed in the context of testing students in classroom subjects such as physics or math. Covering only one aspect of elementary physics might have resulted in the conclusion that the test lacked content validity. As the field of psychometrics grew, those concerned with data collection instruments in fields other than education began to apply this concept to the measurement of other behaviors, attitudes, skills, or types of knowledge.

3. *Criterion-related validity*: Another kind of validity asks if there is agreement between the responses to this instrument and some other measure obtained independently by the same subjects. For example, is there a high positive correlation between the total score on the Graduate Record Exam (GRE) and another measure of aptitude for graduate-level coursework, such as the undergraduate grade point average (GPA)? If there is, then the GRE might be said to be the gold standard in this psychometric study, and the variable being used in this study (the GPA) is said to have criterion-related validity.

4. *Construct validity*: A construct is a theory or representation of a concept, and this type of validity asks whether the data collection instrument clearly represents that theory. For example, the construct *quality of care* needs to be clearly defined in order to develop a data collection instrument about such care. If the instrument is an accurate representation of such an abstract concept, then it is said to have construct validity.

Reliability

Instrument reliability is basically concerned with stability over time and testing conditions. For example, if we ask a subject to rate her level of pain on a 10-point scale at 2 separate points in time *under the same circumstances*, and if there is no change in her condition, then we should expect to get approximately the same ratings. If so, then the data collection instrument (in this case, one question about rating pain) can be said to have instrument reliability.

> Think of the data collection instrument as a ruler. If the ruler is made of a material that does not vary because of the surrounding temperature (for example, it doesn't expand with heat or shrink with extreme cold), and it is always accurate regardless of the conditions or if the material does not become fatigued with age, then the ruler can be said to be stable. It must be capable of providing reliable measurements.
>
> If we are trying to measure something, such as human behavior, we want the data collection instrument itself to not be subject to change if the subject's behavior did not change. The instrument itself has to be stable.

One of the ways to assess instrument reliability is to conduct a test–retest analysis of the instrument itself. After developing an instrument, such as a survey about the adequacy of drug reimbursement coverage under Medicaid, ask a group of program recipients to respond to the survey (the *test*), wait a short period of time (long enough for them to forget how they responded to each question but not so long that current events or circumstances lead to an actual change), then ask them to fill out the same survey again (the *retest*). If there is a high positive correlation between the responses, then the data collection instrument is said to have a strong test–retest reliability. Note that this test–retest analysis is not the actual research study.

Establishing the validity and reliability of a data collection instrument, especially in a study with primary source data collection, requires time and resources and is not to be undertaken lightly. If researchers can use a data collection instrument that already has validity and reliability reported by others and measures something important in their own study, then they should use it rather than develop their own.

Other Instrument Characteristics

Other basic characteristics of a data collection instrument might include the number of items or questions or the average time needed to gather the information from or about subjects. If the instrument was a survey, note whether the data were collected by mail, telephone, online, or through social media.

Standardized Instruments

If the instruments were standardized, what references are given about this standardization? What normative groups were used in the original standardization, and did the subjects in this study have the same or similar characteristics as those in the normative group? For example, the standardization of a questionnaire about food preferences may have been based on responses from people living in rural Minnesota, but such normative responses might not be appropriate for a study of food preferences of Chinese Americans living in San Francisco.

Some journals permit the author to publish an author-developed survey and its psychometric characteristics (e.g., validity and reliability measures) as an appendix at the end of the journal article; if such a survey has been included, indicate this in your review of the study.

Setting

If it is relevant to the area of research being reviewed, record information about the setting in which the data were collected, for example, urban or rural, community, hospital, nursing home, home, or school. Sometimes the setting can also include measures such as level of poverty or home ownership, as gathered from census records or other data sets.

Not all studies will include every topic mentioned here, and other studies may describe additional topics. Some studies will provide references for the description of the validity and reliability of the instrument or the psychometric characteristics. But in your review of the literature, you will probably be able to determine what kind of instrument was used (questionnaire, interview protocol), what the setting was (in a hospital or the community), and whether some or all of the data were primary or secondary source data. These topics were provided as a guide for examining data collection in a study.

What Are the Results of the Statistical Analysis?

After data collection has been completed, researchers should have the information they need to conduct the statistical analysis. As shown in **Figure 2-9**, the **statistical analysis** section is where researchers describe the statistical tests used and the results of the analysis. There are many kinds of statistical tests, and the field is growing every day. Methods change rapidly, and unless you are a biostatistician, you are not likely to know all of the analytical procedures.

A basic statistics textbook is a good resource for providing background material for this section. The classic book by Siegel on nonparametric statistics is also useful.[11] Statistical methods commonly used in the epidemiological literature include those described in books by Fleiss[12] and Kahn and Sempos.[13]

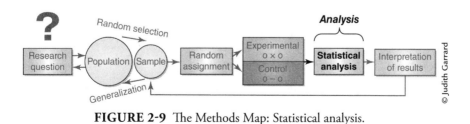

FIGURE 2-9 The Methods Map: Statistical analysis.

As you review the literature, it is important to read the statistical sections of a paper, including the tables describing the characteristics of subjects and the results of differences between the experimental and control groups, but do not assume that you will know about the most recent tests or their appropriate use. Do not get so overwhelmed about the statistical tests and results that you fail to complete your analysis of the paper or complete your review of the literature.

A Philosophy about Statistics

I have a philosophy about statistics that has served me well in conducting reviews of the literature. At the most fundamental level, statistics is a sophisticated set of methods for transforming a lot of information into quantitative data that can be better managed to answer the research questions. It is important for researchers to make the statistical summaries meaningful and the results understandable to the reader, but sometimes these explanations are not meaningful enough. Your goal in reviewing the literature is to always keep your focus on answering the research questions. As you read each study, state the purpose(s) of the study in question form, and those questions will guide you in thinking about the kinds of answers the statistical analysis needs to address.

As you analyze each study, be aware that additional questions may appear. Ask yourself whether the authors provided an answer to a research question that they did not ask initially. Did some results creep into the paper without an explicit research question being described? Were these additional research questions appropriate to the study? A transition from one research question or purpose to another can sometimes be detected in the results section of a paper or in the discussion section. Such a change may occur because the authors allowed the statistically significant results to dictate the hypothesis rather than the other way around. Alternatively, the results to the first question may logically lead to posing and answering a second question. Differences between initial and later research questions may be important to note in a review of the study.

What Is the Interpretation of Results?

As shown in **Figure 2-10**, researchers need to describe their **interpretation of the results** of the statistical analysis. Hopefully this will take the form of stating

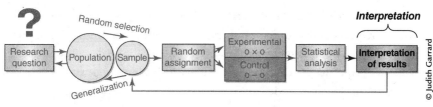

FIGURE 2-10 The Methods Map: Interpretation of results.

the research questions, providing the results, and drawing a reasonable set of interpretations.

If there is no mention of the research questions at this point in the study, then you as the reviewer should conduct that three-part review yourself: state the question, describe the answers based on the statistical analysis, and examine the authors' interpretations. As a reviewer, it is your role to decide whether the authors' interpretations are logical and valid, based on the results of the study. You must also decide whether the results of the study are consistent with the findings of other studies on the same topic, as described elsewhere in the literature. Did the authors describe the strengths and weaknesses of the study? Did they address issues such as whether the findings could be generalized, problems with methodological design that were present but could not have been remedied, sample size adequacy, or sampling design?

> Authors who do not point out the weaknesses of their own studies make themselves vulnerable to such criticisms from others. Most authors are pleased to describe the strengths of their studies; some may be reluctant to discuss the weaknesses.

As you review each paper, note whether the conclusions and the significance of the findings related to the results. Do you agree with those conclusions? Bear in mind that statistical significance does not always result in clinical significance or a meaningful impact.

Data Visualization

Until recently most authors of peer-reviewed papers in the health sciences used graphs, histograms, or pie charts to provide additional understanding of the statistical results and their interpretation. With growing use of the Internet, new tools have been developed that can better communicate the authors' interpretation of research findings to the reader. This set of tools can be described as data visualization. Appendix C describes how data visualization can be used in research studies and in literature reviews of those research papers now and in the future. To access Appendix C, use the access code at the front of your book.

Data visualization can be used by authors to tell a story about what the results mean. It is their interpretation. Data visualization is not the only way to provide an interpretation, but it is one of the newer tools available to the research community and will probably become more useful in the future, and that is why Appendix C should be of interest to you as you review the literature.

Who Do the Results of the Study Apply To?

Now look at the **arrow** in **Figure 2-11** that goes from the **interpretation of results** back to the **sample** of subjects. What this arrow means is that the statistical results and interpretation are applicable to the **sample** (i.e., all of the original subjects the researchers began with) and then back through the chain to the **population** (but only if researchers used **random selection of subjects** in the population to form the sample). This application of results to the population is known as **generalization** to the population. From there, researchers use the results and interpretations to answer the **research question** they began with. As you review the literature, record for each study whether the results and interpretation were applicable to the population or the sample.

No Random Sample

Who do the results apply to if the researchers did not use random sampling? Remember the two-way bridge described in Figure 2-3? At the beginning of the study, if researchers have not crossed over the bridge from the population to

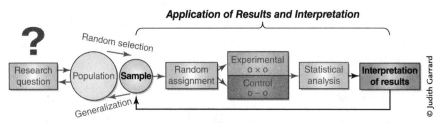

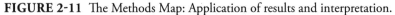

FIGURE 2-11 The Methods Map: Application of results and interpretation.

create a random sample, then at the end of the study they cannot cross back over the bridge from the sample to the population when they are ready to apply the results and interpretation to the research question.

Without random sampling, the results and interpretation are applicable only to the sample. Is this a serious limitation of the study? Not necessarily. Most research studies involving human subjects in the health sciences peer-reviewed literature are not able to draw a random sample from the population because they cannot gain access to the entire population.

Randomized Control Trial

In reviewing the literature, you will find that some authors use the terms *randomized controlled trial* or *randomized clinical trial* or *RCT* (which can cover either).

In a study with an RCT design, the researchers randomly assign subjects to groups (experimental and control) before the intervention is applied. How they

Here is an example. Researchers asked the question, Do women delivering babies rate their quality of health care experience better when delivered by nurse–midwives compared to gynecologists? The sample of subjects was women having babies. The independent variable had two attributes: nurse–midwives (experimental group) and gynecologists (control group). The dependent variable was the rating scale, Quality of Healthcare Experience Outcomes, which the subjects filled out postdelivery.

In this study it was not possible to generate a random sample throughout the United States from all women who were having babies. Nor was it feasible to define the population as all women in a geographic region within a health care system that had multiple hospitals. To make this study practical, with reasonable costs, the researchers recruited women who were delivering within one hospital who agreed to participate. The recruitment period was for 6 months. Subjects were randomly assigned to the experimental or control groups, which meant the women could not choose whether they were cared for by a nurse–midwife or a gynecologist. This is an example of a study with no random sample from the population but with random assignment to groups. Such a study can still make a valuable contribution to the literature.

did this random assignment or how complex the process was may or may not be described in the paper. An RCT (or its equivalent in the behavioral sciences, a classical experimental design) can make an important contribution to the scientific literature, but an RCT says nothing about generalization to the population. If the authors of a study with an RCT design did not initially generate a random sample from the population, they could not generalize their results back to the population after the analysis was completed.

As you review the literature, you will become more proficient in understanding the studies you analyze and will be more able to walk in the footsteps of the researchers. These guidelines and the Methods Map describe an overview of research methods and options available to researchers and guidance for those who conduct reviews of the health sciences peer-reviewed literature.

Here are two examples of studies in the literature in which there was no random selection of subjects for the sample, but there was random assignment of subjects in the sample to the experimental and control groups.

One frequently cited study was based on a sample of subjects in 40 clinical centers in the United States. This was a very large study that had a major impact on choices that women made about their health.[14]

In another RCT, 70 subjects were randomly assigned to the experimental group (with a 50% reduction in TV and computer use) or the control group (with no restriction on access to TV and computer time).[15]

Read both of these papers and discuss with others to understand what the results were. This exercise will help you as you conduct your own review of the literature.

Caroline's Quest: Learning the Concepts

"So," Caroline looked at Professor Dickerson somewhat challengingly, "isn't the Matrix Method just a spreadsheet that's called a review matrix?"

"No," he replied, "there's more to it than that. The Matrix Method is a system for how you can access, integrate, and use information from a variety of sources to prepare a written synthesis of the scientific literature. In the past, researchers could keep up with the current literature by reading several journals or monitoring the work of a few well-known scientists in a field, or they could simply call or write their friends who did research in that area."

"What's wrong with doing that now?" Caroline asked. This business of accessing and integrating and so forth was beginning to sound rather time consuming as she thought about all the other things she had to do to get her thesis completed. She asked, "Why bother with the Matrix Method?"

Professor Dickerson looked over the top of his glasses at her and said dryly, "Because the amount of scientific literature and the sophistication in the field of research synthesis have grown tremendously. It's rarely possible to develop a comprehensive understanding about the research literature on a topic by using such informal methods. Fortunately, more advanced tools for searching and accessing the literature have become available over the past decade or so. The Matrix Method takes advantage of those tools."

"But no one else in my program has to go to all this trouble for their lit reviews," Caroline complained. Her voice verged on the edge of a whine as she continued, "They just go to the Web, read a few papers, and write up a summary. Takes them several hours at most."

Professor Dickerson nodded his head, "Yes, anyone can do a sloppy job, Caroline." He looked squarely at her. "But they run the risk of not understanding the literature—neither the depth nor the full scope of what's out there. Furthermore, they could miss some of the more important articles or even major trends in a field of research. It is also the case that whatever they write, whether it's a thesis, a scientific paper, or a report about research on a particular topic, has to withstand the scrutiny of readers who are likely to know the literature quite well . . . like your thesis committee members."

Caroline's eyes were beginning to glaze over as he continued, "The person who does a cursory literature review could find himself doing what he thinks is original research, only to discover at the end that that very study was already done and reported by someone else."

Professor Dickerson's enthusiasm began to build. "The process of doing a thorough review of the literature is analogous to solving a mystery. If you miss some of the important clues, then you may not ever find out who or what was responsible for the crime—or what the study really meant, in this case. The

---

EXHIBIT 2-5 Outline of Caroline's Master Folder for Her Thesis

Paper Trail Folder
- Key words
- Key sources
- Electronic bibliographic database
- Internet
- Notes

Documents Folder

Review Matrix Folder

Synthesis Folder

Matrix Method gives you an organized way to lay out all of the pieces and put the puzzle together."

He looked at her with a grin. "The effort will pay off for you, Caroline. You'll see. Now, let's get started."

Under Professor Dickerson's direction, Caroline created a Master Folder on the desktop of her computer and assigned four folders to the Master Folder. She further subdivided the first folder, Paper Trail, into five parts, with one document, to begin with, for each part. The different sections and subsections of Caroline's Master Folder are shown in **Exhibit 2-5**.

Caroline then went to the biomedical library to begin looking up some reference books on smoking behavior. In her opinion, just using Google to search for the topic would have been sufficient, but Professor Dickerson insisted that she read from the original textbooks as her first step.

What You Should Know or Be Able to Do by the End of This Chapter

Chapter 2 is a mini-tutorial about (1) finding what you need in a typical scientific paper and (2) applying what you learned in this chapter about methodological reviews to each of the papers you abstract in using the Matrix Method. The fundamental requirement by the end of Chapter 2 is for you to have gained some experience in reading six or more research papers in your area of interest and conducting a methodological review in each of those six papers.

> ### Hint
>
> Unless this assignment is required as part of a class, you can form a study group of your own, consisting of about three to five colleagues who are also using this book. Agree on the choice of only one set of six papers that all of you will use. Select the first paper, and then all read it and fill in the responses to the first assignment independently. Discuss *at that point* each item in the first assignment and determine what the correct answer should be. Repeat this activity for each of the remaining six papers.
>
> Now go to the second assignment, using the same six papers. Take the first paper, record your responses to a review of the methodological design, and discuss your answers in your group; then do that for each of the other five papers.

Here's what you need to do:

First Assignment: The Anatomy of a Scientific Paper

Your goal in this exercise is to become comfortable with knowing where you can find what you need in a paper. Select six studies on a topic of interest to you, all from different journals.

1. Outline the first paper by the eight sections under the Anatomy of a Scientific Paper as described in this chapter. Specifically describe the following:
   a. Title and Authorship Section. Fill in the title and authorship of the first paper
   b. Abstract Section. In your own words, summarize the abstract here in about three sentences or less describing the purpose of the paper, the methods used, the results, and the authors' conclusions.
   c. Introduction Section. Answer each of the four questions about this paper from the Introduction Section:
      (1) Did the authors describe their own literature review? *Your response:* yes/no
      (2) Did the authors describe why they did this study, that is, their motivation for the study, if so, what was it? *Your response:* yes/no

(3) Did the authors describe the scientific theory or conceptual model that the research was based on in this study? *Your response:* yes/no

(4) Did they describe the purpose of the study? What were their specific research questions (list them)? *Your response:* State each question very specifically; you will be coming back to 1c(4) later in this analysis!

d. Methods Section. For each of the authors' research questions, as stated in 1c(4), answer each of the questions:

(1) Methodological Design

(a) Did the authors use random selection to create a sample in this study? *Your response:* yes/no

(b) What methodological design was used in this study? *Your response:* Describe the type of methodological design used in each question in 1c(4), Behavioral sciences designs: experimental, quasi-experimental, preexperimental, observational, or epidemiological designs: RCT or observational designs (choose one) cohort, case-control, or cross-sectional.

(c) What were the independent and dependent variables (if there was not an independent variable, then say so)? *Your response:* Describe an independent/dependent variable for each question in 1c(4).

(d) Did the authors use random assignment to create two or more groups of subjects? *Your response:* yes/no

(2) Subjects

(a) How many subjects did the study begin with, how many were in the final analysis? *Your response:* State these two numbers.

(b) Did the authors describe any comparisons of the subjects between those who remained in the study and those who dropped out? *Your response:* yes/no

(3) Data Sources

(a) Did the authors use primary source data, that is, did the authors collect the data from the subjects themselves? *Your response:* yes/no

(b) Did the authors use secondary source data? *Your response:* yes/no

(4) Data Collection Methods. Did the authors use any questionnaires or surveys or other data collection methods? *Your response:* yes/no

(5) Statistical and Analytical Procedures. Did the authors describe the statistical or analytical procedures? *Your response:* yes/no. Hint: Look at the titles of the tables or figures they presented and see if the procedure is described.

e. Results Section

(1) Were the results for each research question described in 1c(4)? *Your response:* yes/no

f. Discussion and Conclusion Section

(1) Did the authors summarize the research study? *Your response:* yes/no

g. Did the authors answer each of the research questions they asked in 1c(4)? *Your response:* yes/no

(1) Did authors provide an interpretation and discussion about what the results meant? *Your response:* yes/no

(2) Did the authors describe the strengths and weaknesses of this study? *Your response:* yes/no

(3) Was there any discussion about future research? *Your response:* yes/no

(4) Did the authors say what the significance of the study was, i.e., what impact did it have on clinical practice? *Your response:* yes/no

h. List of References. Glance over the references. Do you see any studies you might add to your review of the literature when you get there? *Your response:* yes/no

i. Acknowledgments Section. Did the authors say where they got the funding for this research? *Your response:* yes/no

j. Do you detect any sense of conflict between those who funded it and what the conclusions were? *Your response:* yes/no

Having done that for the first paper you chose, go back and fill out the same information for the second paper. Now complete the rest of this assignment one paper at a time. With experience, this assignment will be very quickly accomplished by the time you finish the sixth paper. By then you should know at a fundamental level how a scientific paper is organized.

This was essentially a scavenger hunt, with mostly yes/no answers. Note how the answers may vary based on the particular journal, or by papers within a journal. This is an important part of learning where things are in a scientific paper.

Second Assignment: A Methodological Review
Using the Methods Map

With the second assignment, you will use the same six papers in your area of interest and conduct a methodological review using the 11 versions of the Methods Map in Chapter 2. This will be a different and more in-depth review, and one essential to your training in how to conduct a literature review in later chapters in this book.

Hint

Since you will be using your own version of the Methods Map in this assignment, you might want to make six copies (one for each study) of Figure 2-1 The Methods Map, then use that copy for modifying the first study based on your answers to the following eleven questions. You will need to look at the specific figure of the Methods Map to respond to each question, but you can record your answers on one sheet for Figure 2-1 per study. Repeat for each of the six studies.

Using the Methods Map, take the first paper and answer these questions:

1. Figure 2-1 The Methods Map
   a. Read the first paper again, then do this: Map only *one* of the questions in 1(c)4 for this paper. *Your response:* Lay out Figure 2-1 in a Methods Map that reflects this study. You may need to fill this out later as you progress through the next 10 variations of the Methods Map. If so, then return to this first question and modify the Methods Map based on your study.
2. Figure 2-2 The Methods Map: Purpose of the Study
   a. What was the first research question? *Your response:* On the same page below the Methods Map, state only the first research question briefly in one or two sentences. You will need to refer back to that research question as you complete this assignment; having it in a convenient place will help.
3. Figure 2-3 The Methods Map: Population and Sample
   a. Did the authors have access to a population, and then did they use random selection to draw a sample from that population? *Your response:*

Change the Methods Map to indicate this. If no population was used, put an X through the Population arrow. Likewise, put an X through the Random Selection arrow if you did not know how the sample was obtained or if the subjects were recruited by some means other than random sampling.

4. Figure 2-4 The Methods Map: Subjects in Sample
   a. How many subjects were in the original sample? *Your response:* State the number or "I cannot tell."
   b. Did the authors include each of the following in their description of the sample: unit of analysis, inclusion/exclusion criteria for defining an eligible subject, number of subjects in final analysis, and subject characteristics (such as age, gender, race/ethnicity, geographic area, above/below poverty line, etc.)? *Your response:* List each of these four characteristics and put yes/no beside each one after you have read this section. (Hint: Also check the end of the paper in the analysis section to see if the answers to some these questions are given there.)

5. Figure 2-5 The Methods Map: Random Assignment of Subjects to Groups
   a. Did the authors use random assignment of subjects in the sample to groups? If no, put an X over Random Assignment in your version of the Methods Map. If yes, then don't modify your version of the Map. How many groups were in this study (for this first research question)? *Your response:* Modify your version of the Map to show the number of groups.

6. Figure 2-6 The Methods Map: Random Selection and Random Assignment
   a. Did this study have both random selection and random assignment or was only one of these decisions made? Reread the section in the book titled, "How Do Random Selection and Random Assignment Differ?" *Your response:* Put an X (if one does not already exist) over Random Selection if that was not used and over Random Assignment if that was not used.

7. Figure 2-7 The Methods Map: Independent and Dependent Variables
   a. In the authors' discussion of the study, did they state what the independent variables were? *Your response:* Draw an arrow to the independent variable on your version of the Map (see Figure 2-7 for guidance), write "independent variable" and state above that label what the variable was. If there was no independent variable in the first question (from 1c(4)), then put an X through Independent Variable on your version of the Map.

b. Did the authors describe at least one dependent variable? *Your response:* Show with an arrow(s) where the dependent variable was in this study and state beneath the label what that dependent variable was. Hint: You can't put an X over the dependent variable. There *always* has to be a dependent variable in a study. Always!

8. Figure 2-8 The Methods Map: Data Collection
   a. Describe the following about the data collection instrument and procedures:

      Were primary, secondary, or both sources of data used?

      Your response: Primary source data collection: yes/no

      Secondary source data collection: yes/no

      Combination of both: yes/no

9. Figure 2-9 The Methods Map: Statistical Analysis
   a. What was at least one of the statistical analysis procedures done in this study? *Your response:* Write the name of the statistical analysis procedure above the words "Statistical Analysis" in your version of the Map.

10. Figure 2-10. The Methods Map: Interpretation of Results
    a. Did the authors discuss the meaning of the statistical results? *Your response:* Write in what section of the paper the authors describe this. Put your response above the words, "Interpretation of Results" in your version of the Map.
    b. Did the authors report strengths *and* weaknesses of this study? *Your response:* yes/no (if only one, e.g., strengths but not weaknesses, then a "yes" is not appropriate).

11. Figure 2-11 The Methods Map: Application of Results and Interpretation
    a. To whom did the authors apply the results? *Your response:* If the sample is correctly represented in Figure 2-11, then leave the arrow in your version of the Map unmarked; if there was no mention of who the results applied to, then put an X through the arrow.
    b. Did the authors apply the results to the population? *Your response:* If yes *and* if they used random selection from the population to create a sample, then draw a dotted line from the sample to the population. If they generalized (inappropriately) from the sample to the population, with no random selection at the beginning of the study or if there was an X through the population, then create the same dotted line on your version of the map and put an X in the middle of it.

Now repeat this set of questions with each of the remaining studies, one study at a time, using a new copy of Figure 2-1 The Methods Map. Upon completion of this second assignment, you should be well equipped to proceed to the next chapter of this book!

REFERENCES

1. Garrard J, Cooper SL, Goertz C. Drug use management in board and care facilities. *Gerontologist.* 1997; 37(6):748-756.
2. Strunk W, White EB. *The Elements of Style.* 4th ed. New York: Longman Publisher; 1999.
3. American Psychological Association. *Publication Manual of the American Psychological Association.* 4th ed. Washington, DC: American Psychological Association; 1994.
4. Iverson C. *American Medical Association Manual of Style: A Guide for Authors and Editors.* 9th ed. Baltimore, MD: Williams & Wilkins; 1998.
5. Krueger RA. *Focus Groups: A Practical Guide for Applied Research.* Thousand Oaks, CA: Sage Publications; 1994.
6. Campbell DT, Stanley JC. *Experimental and Quasi-experimental Designs for Research.* Chicago, IL: Rand McNally; 1966.
7. Cook TD, Campbell DT. *Quasi-experimentation: Design and Analysis Issues for Field Settings.* Chicago, IL: Rand McNally; 1979.
8. Kleinbaum DG, Kupper LL, Morgenstern H. *Epidemiologic Research: Principles and Quantitative Methods.* New York: Van Nostrand Reinhold; 1982.
9. Salant P, Dilman DA. *How to Conduct Your Own Survey.* New York: John Wiley & Sons; 1994.
10. Dillman DA. *Mail and Telephone Surveys: The Total Design Method.* New York: John Wiley & Sons; 1978.
11. Siegel S, Castellan NJ Jr. *Nonparametric Statistics for the Behavioral Sciences.* 2nd ed. New York: McGraw-Hill Higher Education; 1989.
12. Fleiss JL. *Statistical Methods for Rates and Proportions.* New York: John Wiley & Sons; 1981.
13. Kahn HA, Sempos CT. Statistical methods in epidemiology. In: *Monographs in Epidemiology and Biostatistics.* Vol. 12. New York: Oxford University Press; 1989.
14. Anderson GL, Limacher M, Assaf AR, et al. Effects of conjugated equine estrogen in postmenopausal women with hysterectomy: The Women's Health Initiative randomized controlled trial. *JAMA.* 2004;291(14):1701-1712.
15. Epstein LH, Roemmich JN, Robinson JL, et al. A randomized trial of the effects of reducing television viewing and computer use on body mass index in young children. *Arch Pediatr Adolesc Med.* 2008;162(3):239-245.

PART II

The Matrix Method

The Matrix Method is described in Chapters 3 through 6. Each of the four chapters covers different aspects of the Matrix Method, but all are necessary in successfully writing a synthesis of the literature. Each chapter discusses one of the four major folders: Paper Trail Folder, Documents Folder, Review Matrix Folder, and Synthesis Folder.

Despite their differences in content, the four chapters have several themes in common, including:

- a description of the purpose of the chapter,
- the definition of the title of the folder, with one or more examples,
- an outline of the topics covered in the chapter,
- a section on how to organize the folder or subfolder,
- explanations about how to assemble and use the contents of each folder,
- Caroline's Quest, which describes the process of applying what you have learned in the chapter, and
- What You Should Know or Be Able to Do by the End of This Chapter.

CHAPTER 3

Paper Trail Folder: How to Plan and Manage a Search of the Literature

This chapter is about how to set up and use a paper trail and how to organize and conduct a search for source materials. This will be the most useful to you in the beginning stages of your literature review. The six sections of this chapter are the following:

- What Is a Paper Trail?
- How to Organize a Paper Trail Folder
- Resources for Creating and Using a Paper Trail
- Tips on Searching for Source Documents
- Caroline's Quest: Managing the Search
- What You Should Know or Be Able to Do by the End of This Chapter

WHAT IS A PAPER TRAIL?

In the Matrix Method, the Paper Trail Folder is a place to record lists, notes, websites, and a description of anything else that helped you to plan and keep track of what you have done as you review the literature on a particular topic. This is also a place for you to document your search for relevant materials.

Advantages of a Paper Trail

A paper trail is both a map of where you are going and a diary of where you have been in your search for source documents. The map gets you started and buys you efficiency; the diary helps you remember what you have done so that you can avoid redoing the same thing. Think of the paper trail as a personal blog (to yourself) about the process. Even people with a prodigious memory will find themselves backtracking and trying to relocate materials if they have not taken time to make a list of the sources explored and the articles considered. It is also useful to write down the names of people who were (or were not) helpful. A knowledgeable and enthusiastic librarian can be worth his or her weight in gold—record the person's name for future reference. The same advice applies to helpful faculty and colleagues.

HOW TO ORGANIZE A PAPER TRAIL FOLDER

Just as you unfold a map as the first step in going on a hike in unfamiliar territory, the first step in beginning a review of the literature should be to set up a Paper Trail Folder, which is the first of the four folders in the Master Folder; the others are the Documents Folder, the Review Matrix Folder, and the Synthesis Folder. In the past, index cards were traditionally used in conducting a review of the literature, but now, they are irrelevant since literature reviews (and the Matrix Method) are based on a computer.

How to Organize a Paper Trail Folder

The Paper Trail Folder has five subfolders: (1) Key Words Subfolder, (2) Resources Subfolder, (3) Bibliographic Databases Subfolder, (4) Internet Documents Subfolder, and (5) Miscellaneous Notes Subfolder. The Paper Trail Folder is essentially your filing cabinet, and the subfolders are the file drawers where you can store specific information. Create the subfolders now as you begin to use the Matrix Method. Here is the function of each of the subfolders:

1. **Key Words Subfolder**. A *key word* is a term or phase that describes a research topic. In a word processing document, generate and store a list of key words that you have identified and others that you have considered but discarded and put that document in your Key Words Subfolder. Begin the key words document by typing the purpose of the literature review at the top of the page. Think of the words that describe that topic.

For example, if this is a review of the literature on the epidemiology of pneumonia of elderly in nursing hones, some of the key words might be *pneumonia, nursing homes,* and *elderly.*

The key words that you record will be useful when you set the parameters for searching the literature. As you collect information during the review of the literature, add to this list. Some of the terms you considered initially may not be useful as the literature review progresses. Leave these terms on the list, but enter a strikethrough or otherwise mark them differently—it is useful to know which terms did not work and as well as those that did.

2. **Resources Subfolder**. In the Resources Subfolder, you can store notes about the names of reference books, journals, government reports, and other materials that you considered or reviewed. This is also the place to record the names of people who have helped you (or not) in your process of doing a literature review. The same logic of maintaining a list of where you are going and where you have been applies to all of the library sources considered or explored. For example, create separate word processing documents in the Resources Subfolder. One document will be a list of reference books, other books, journals, and other print sources; the other will be a list of helpful people. Create as many documents as you need to make this Subfolder easy to use.

3. **Bibliographic Databases Subfolder**. In the Bibliographic Databases Subfolder, make a list of electronic databases used, such as MEDLINE, CINAHL, and PsycINFO. Then create one word processing document for each database, and in each document, record the following:

   What was the date of the search? Put this at the top of the page, and again each time you create a new search. Then for each search with this database, record the following:
   • What key words did you use?
   • What restrictions did you place on the search, e.g., English language journals only or review articles only (or both)?
   • What period of time did you cover, e.g., 2010 to the present.

   When you have completed the search, copy and paste the entire search strategy (the instructions you gave to do the search) on this page in the Bibliographic Databases Subfolder. Then repeat this procedure every time you do another search.

4. **Internet Documents Subfolder**. When researching on the Web, it is easy to lose track of what has been explored unless you keep a record. Maintain

a list of the Internet documents you examined in this subfolder, the date accessed, search restrictions such as date range (e.g., 1995 to 2015), and brief notes on information obtained. Also, set bookmarks in your browser for commonly used websites. Another possibility is to copy the URL of the home page of useful websites and store this information on a separate page (perhaps titled, Useful Websites) in this Internet Documents Subfolder.

5. **Miscellaneous Notes Subfolder**. Treat this subfolder like a collection of miscellaneous notes (i.e., a diary of things that you need to remember). Use a page each to describe where to find hard-to-locate materials, for example, "*Journal of Scientific Wonder* is located in the third stack from the left in the basement of the library of the county medical examiner." The notes refer to the search process, not the papers themselves. Store those notes in this subfolder.

This Miscellaneous Notes Subfolder can also be used to store notes about additional references of scientific papers or other materials discovered in the process of looking at other sources. Put a check mark by each as you skimmed the content and accepted or discarded the paper. In recording a reference, use a standard format, such as APA or AMA style, to make sure you have all the information you need, including publisher, date of publication, and page numbers. Inevitably, the one article without the year of publication will be the very one that is essential in writing your synthesis of the literature. It is best to be consistent in the first place.

Record All Authors

In recording a reference to a paper in a journal, consider the following tip. Scientific journals are expensive to produce, and editors are inclined to be stingy with space. One way some publishers save space in the references section of a book or journal article is to restrict the names of multiple authors to the first three individuals followed by "et al." for the remaining authors. In reviewing these papers, however, you might want to depart from this protocol by consistently writing down the names of all of the authors in recording references in the Paper Trail Folder and especially later in the Review Matrix Folder. There is a practical reason for doing this.

In many fields of study, the research is conducted jointly by a number of scientists. Although the first author of a paper presumably had the most responsibility for writing the paper or doing the study, some of the other authors may have been publishing in the field over a longer period of time. These more established scientists sometimes are listed by choice as last in the authorship.

Alternatively, authors of some large, well-established research teams have chosen to list their names alphabetically, signifying equal importance in the contribution of all members of the research team to the study. With either practice, there can be a problem in tracking the work of specific individuals if the format of the reference is limited to the first three authors followed by "et al." Consider recording all of the authors' names; usually they are listed on the paper itself. After the Paper Trail Folder is set up, you are ready to begin your search of the literature.

Clarifying Incomplete Citations

There will come a point, usually at the end of your patience or right before a deadline, when you will come upon one of your citations that is missing a crucial piece of information, such as a date or volume number. PubMed may have a solution for this problem. Copy the following paragraph, save in a Word document, and store in your Internet Documents Subfolder.

Go to the PubMed home page (http://www.ncbi.nlm.nih.gov/pubmed/citmatch). Under PubMed Tools, select Single Citation Matcher. At the resulting site, you can type in any information that you have about the citation (you do not even have to have the exact title), and PubMed will try to provide you with one or more options that fit your criteria. This is a nifty tool whether you have run out of time or not!

RESOURCES FOR CREATING AND USING A PAPER TRAIL

The Reference Librarian: An Essential Resource for Your Literature Review

Your most important resource in the beginning stages of your literature review is the professional at your university library whose title is usually "reference librarian." Your interaction with this person will be all the more valuable if you first read over the rest of this chapter. The reference librarian will use many of the terms described here, and you will have a head start by already knowing what these terms mean.

What can you expect from the reference librarian? He or she will begin by asking you what the purpose of your literature review is, what question(s) you want to answer, and what your deadline is. Create a Word document every time you meet with him or her. Record his or her name, telephone number, e-mail address, and the date of each interaction, whether in person or by phone or e-mail. Take copious notes and store each of these documents in your Resources Subfolder.

At this first session, the reference librarian may show you how to do an online search, probably using PubMed. Take more notes or ask for a handout which you can digitally scan and save in the Resources Subfolder.

Get a copy of that preliminary search and note the total number of references he or she finds. This is the first step in eventually filling out the PRISMA Flowchart[1] of Documents in your review of the literature (see Chapter 1). You will report the final copy of this flowchart, complete with numbers from your searches, in the final synthesis of your review. You will probably modify this computer run several times in the future.

Each time you make a new PubMed run, record the instructions and the limits. These limits are often in the form of key words and the inclusions/exclusions of the studies. For example, what time period did you put around your review (e.g., from 2000–2015)? Or what inclusions did you apply to the studies, e.g., English language only, or exclusions, such as no editorials, or opinion pieces, or marketing materials? Ask the reference librarian what else would be appropriate to exclude.

Better yet, ask if there is a class available (for free) at the library on how to use PubMed. Take it. At some point, he or she may also ask which reference management software, such as RefWorks or EndNote, you are using. If that set of skills is absent in your repertoire, then sign up for the class. Often, the software is available free to registered students at the university.

Clearly this interaction will have to start very early in the process of your literature review. If you skip the reference librarian, then you will be behind the game the whole way. If you start too late, then you are unlikely to make your deadline. He or she is absolutely the most important person in these initial stages. Return to the reference librarian or his or her counterpart every time you can. There may be more than one reference librarian; record all their names. Their job is to help you learn how this works and identify the skills you need to get this done effectively and efficiently.

Now, here is what you should learn before you go to see the reference librarian.

Reference Books: Learn Something about the Topic

If you are not familiar with the topic or subject of the literature you are reviewing, it is important to take time to learn some of the fundamental information about the disease or issue. Reference books can be especially useful resources at the beginning of a review of the literature in providing an overview of the topic and a potential list of key words. In a biomedical library, these books are often kept on reserve and therefore are readily available. Check with a librarian about the major reference books on the topic you want to review. For example, if you are reviewing the literature on pharmaceutical treatment of arthritis, consult a basic medical textbook about arthritic conditions and their treatments before embarking on a review of the research literature on arthritis medications.

As you consult a reference book or textbook, develop a list of key words, including the terms those authors used. Keep this information in the Key Words Subfolder. Maintain a list of the textbooks or reference books examined, and for each book, record references of papers and other books mentioned at the end of chapters that relate to your subject. You might also make a digital scan of these source materials and store them in the Miscellaneous Notes Subfolder.

Record the names of journals cited frequently in these source materials. This list of frequently appearing journals will also be useful in the next step: storing copies of articles from scientific journals in the Source Documents Subfolder.

If you are already familiar with the subject under review, the most efficient approach might be to now make a list of key words for your topic.

Key Words and Controlled Vocabulary: Searching Electronic Databases

In searching for journal articles in most health sciences databases, you can use key words or a controlled vocabulary of key words. Key words are terms that describe the characteristics of a subject you are reviewing. A controlled vocabulary is an organized list of approved terms or key words that indexers of the journal or set of journals used to describe the same journal articles.

Key Words

Key word searching consists of looking for the occurrence of the word(s) in the title or abstract of the article exactly as it is typed in the search box. If the author uses an alternative spelling or synonym for the topic, there is no guarantee that the article will be retrieved by the key word search. For example, if the author used the word *tumor* in the title or abstract, but you used the key word *cancer*, then there is no guarantee that the search will retrieve that article.

Key word searching can be helpful when you are looking for a new drug or a new procedure that has not yet been introduced into the controlled vocabulary of the database. In such a case, key word searching may be the only effective way of retrieving articles about the topic.

Controlled Vocabulary

When you use the controlled vocabulary to search the same journals in the same database, you are using the terms that indexers used when they indexed the articles. The controlled vocabulary in MEDLINE/PubMed is called MeSH (medical subject headings). For example, the official MeSH heading for cancer is the controlled vocabulary term *neoplasms*. It does not matter whether an author uses *cancer* or *tumor* in the text of the article; the use of the controlled vocabulary term will guarantee retrieval of all articles on the topic.

Most databases provide users with direct access to the controlled vocabulary so you can see for yourself whether a given term exists for searching. The U.S. National Library of Medicine provides access to the MeSH database, a list of FAQs, and tutorials at this website: http://www.ncbi.nlm.nih.gov/mesh.

Identifying Controlled Vocabulary in Abstracts

Another way to identify controlled vocabulary terms is to examine the abstracts of articles in electronic bibliographic databases (e.g., MEDLINE, CINAHL). For example, consider the abstract from PubMed shown in **Exhibit 3-1**. Three of the

---

EXHIBIT 3-1   Abstract in the Citation Display from PubMed

Arch Intern Med. 2003 Oct 27;163(19):2290-5.

Variations in product choices of frequently purchased herbs: caveat emptor.

Garrard J, Harms S, Eberly LE, Matiak A.

Divisions of Health Services Research & Policy, School of Public Health, and College of Pharmacy, University of Minnesota, Minneapolis 55455, USA. jgarrard@umn.edu

Abstract

BACKGROUND: Patients who report use of herbs to their physicians may not be able to accurately describe the ingredients or recommended dosage because the products for the same herb may differ. The purpose of this study was to describe variations in label information of products for each of the 10 most commonly purchased herbs.

METHODS: Products for each of 10 herbs were surveyed in a convenience sample of 20 retail stores in a large metropolitan area. Herbs were those with the greatest sales dollars in 1998: echinacea, St John's wort, Ginkgo biloba, garlic, saw palmetto, ginseng, goldenseal, aloe, Siberian ginseng, and valerian.

RESULTS: Each herb had a large range in label ingredients and recommended daily dose (RDD) across available products. Strengths were not directly comparable because of ingredient variability. Among 880 products, 43% were consistent with a benchmark in ingredients and RDD, 20% in ingredients only, and 37% were either not consistent or label information was insufficient. Price per RDD was a significant predictor of consistency with the benchmark, but store type was not.

CONCLUSIONS: Persons self-medicating with an herb may be ingesting ingredients substantially different from that recommended by a benchmark, both in quantity and content. Higher price per label RDD was the best predictor of consistency with a benchmark. This study demonstrates that health providers and consumers need to closely examine label ingredients of presumably the same or similar herbal products.

PMID: 14581247 [PubMed - indexed for MEDLINE]

⊖ **MeSH Terms**

MeSH Terms

Cross-Sectional Studies

Drug Labeling*

Herbal Medicine*

Humans

Plants, Medicinal/chemistry*

Reprinted from PubMed, the National Library of Medicine. Abstract adapted with permission by the American Medical Association, 2006. All rights reserved. Garrard J, Harms S, Eberly LE, Matiak A. Variations in product choices of frequently purchased herbs: caveat emptor. *Arch Intern Med.* 2003;163(19):2290–2295.[2]

five MeSH subject headings have an asterisk: Drug Labeling*; Herbal Medicine*; and Plants, Medicinal/chemistry.* An asterisk indicates that the MeSH subject heading is a major focus of the article. To find other citations that have a primary focus on those topics, restrict your PubMed search to the asterisked MeSH headings by typing the MeSH heading followed by the qualifier "[majr]" in square brackets. For example, type "drug labeling [majr]" to search for citations that have a major focus on drug labeling.

Electronic Bibliographic Databases: Many Options, Many Differences

Although MEDLINE was one of the first major electronic bibliographic databases, numerous other databases that cover different subjects and time periods in the health sciences literature are available, some of which are listed in **Exhibit 3-2**. The major database of clinical medicine, MEDLINE, has been freely available on the Internet since 1997 with the National Library of Medicine's (NLM's) PubMed interface. You will find it very instructive to run the same search, using

EXHIBIT 3-2 Examples of Electronic Bibliographic Databases in the Health Sciences

Database	Dates Covered	Subjects Covered
BIOSIS Previews	1969–present	Biology, biotechnology, biochemistry
CINAHL	1982–present	Nursing and allied health
CURRENT CONTENTS	Period varies	Multidisciplinary
Digital Dissertations	1861–present	Abstracts of doctoral dissertations and masters theses from North American universities
Health and Psychosocial Instruments	1985–present	Measurement instruments in health and behavioral sciences
International Pharmaceutical Abstracts	1970–present	Pharmaceutical science and practice
MEDLINE	1966–present	Health sciences
PsycINFO	1974–present	Psychological literature
Sociological Abstracts	1963–present	Sociological literature

the same key words in two or more of these databases, such as MEDLINE and CINAHL. The databases serve different audiences, and there can be differences in which articles are identified.

After you have generated a list of controlled vocabulary terms and some key words, run a search of the literature in whichever electronic bibliographic database you choose (e.g., MEDLINE/PubMed), even if the list is not complete.

In your initial search of the literature in an electronic database, use a search strategy that is as broad as possible. For example, when specifying the instructions for an electronic search, include all types of source documents, such as editorials or review summaries or letters to the editor, about a particular scientific topic. Even if you do not intend to use such nonempirical communications in your final review of the literature, they may be useful in locating other, more relevant scientific papers that you might not have found otherwise. Editorials and letters to the editor can also be enlightening in suggesting counterpoints or alternative opinions about a study. Finally, these nonempirical communications often include new citations that may be especially useful as you expand your search.

Maintain a copy of database search strategies, that is, the instructions you specify for the electronic search, and the complete list of source materials selected. A practical way to do this is to copy the instructions just before initiating the electronic search and then keep a copy, with the date of the search, in the electronic bibliographic databases document in your Internet Documents Subfolder. This information may be useful when you check the thoroughness of your search or later when you document the search strategy in writing your synthesis of the literature.

A few words of caution: First, conduct the computer search of the literature yourself. This will give you the opportunity to scan a title, consider which authors were involved in the study, or rapidly read the abstract. Such information may be crucial in deciding whether to select the article for further consideration.

In the process of working with the initial results of a computer search, you will begin to pick up subtle cues about what else is in the literature. For example, when scrolling through a list of abstracts by a particular author, you will notice the names of other authors associated with a topic or a journal that often publishes papers in this area. Such information is useful in the later stages of the literature review.

A second cautionary note is to remember that not all journals are included in even the most frequently used databases such as MEDLINE. This is especially true for some of the newer journals or those with a specialized focus. For this reason, it is important to extend your search of the literature to the print versions of some of the scientific journals.

Scientific Journals: The Most Current Research Literature

In this era of electronic information, it is easier than ever to stay current on new research that is about to be published in the scholarly literature. The days of scanning tables of contents or year-end indexes of journals are gone.

PubMed, the NLM's interface to the MEDLINE database, provides access to new research by including publisher-submitted citations to forthcoming articles before publication. These records are indicated in PubMed with the tag "(PubMed—as supplied by publisher)" and can be found in PubMed by searching for a key word, author, or journal title. Publishers can also submit citations that will appear in the electronic (or Web) versions of their publications in advance of the print publication. These citations will appear in PubMed with the tag "(Epub ahead of print)."

Most of these sources will then go through the indexing process and receive a new tag such as "(PubMed-in process)" before being completely indexed for MEDLINE. Not all of these publisher-supplied documents will be indexed for MEDLINE. Other commercial bibliographic database providers of MEDLINE, such as OVID, may include these in-process documents as a separate database. Check with your institution's reference librarian to determine whether you have access to these files.

A fact sheet from the U.S. National Library of Medicine is available that explains in greater detail the differences between MEDLINE, PubMed, and the PubMed Central (PMC) at this website: https://www.nlm.nih.gov/pubs/factsheets /dif_med_pub.html.

Another way to be learn about upcoming publications is to sign up for email alerts directly from the publisher. Many health sciences journals offer this type of service, and it is usually free. If you sign up for these email alert services, you will receive the tables of contents of new issues before publication. For example, by searching for the *Journal of the American Medical Association* (*JAMA*) using Google, you can find the American Medical Association URL, which will offer you the option of free email alerts of tables of content of *JAMA* and *Archives* journals. These include *JAMA*, the *Archives of Dermatology, Facial Plastic Surgery, General Psychiatry, Internal Medicine, Neurology, Ophthalmology, Otolaryngology, Head & Neck Surgery, Pediatrics & Adolescent Medicine*, and *Surgery*. Other journals can be located via Google or another search engine. If all else fails, then ask the reference librarian for help.

Research in Progress: NIH RePORTER

In reviewing the literature, it is sometimes useful to know about studies that are in progress, even if the results are not yet available. For example, if you are thinking about applying for a grant proposal, it is important to find out if a similar study has already been funded. Alternatively, you might have a pressing clinical or patient-related problem for which there is little or no information in the literature, and you need to know who is doing research on that issue. You may want to identify researchers who have not yet published in an area but who might be presenting results at upcoming scientific meetings. By identifying current research projects, you can follow them in future literature or contact the researchers directly about preliminary findings or their plans for publication of results.

Although a list of all research studies ever conducted, or even those currently in progress, does not exist, you can identify many of the research projects funded by the federal government by conducting a search on the NIH RePORTER. The RePORTER (the RePORT Expenditures and Results module) is part of the larger National Institutes of Health (NIH) website, the Research Portfolio Online Reporting Tool (RePORT), at https://projectreporter.nih.gov/reporter.cfm, which was launched in 2009.

The NIH RePORTER is a searchable database of federally funded biomedical research projects conducted at universities, hospitals, and other research institutions. Projects that have been completed and those currently in progress are included in the database. The NIH RePORTER includes studies funded by NIH, the Substance Abuse and Mental Health Services Administration, the Health Resources and Services Administration, the Food and Drug Administration, the Centers for Disease Control and Prevention, the Agency for Healthcare Research and Quality (AHRQ), and Veterans Affairs.

Another resource is ClinicalTrials.gov at this website: http://www.clinicaltrials.gov, which provides information about a registry and a database of human randomized clinical trials that are either in progress or are being initiated. The location and a telephone number are provided for the public if the study is still recruiting subjects. A tutorial is available for using ClinicalTrials.gov at their website.

Government Reports: How to Find Them

Over the past 5 or more years, different health-related agencies of the federal government have begun to provide special reports on the Internet. A free, searchable database of documents printed by the U.S. Government Printing Office (GPO) is available on the Internet at GPO Access. The home page of GPO is http://www.gpo.gov. At that website, click "Catalog of U.S. Government Publications" or go to: http://catalog.gpo.gov/F?RN=945439079.

Discuss with a reference librarian the search procedures for accessing congressional reports and other federal documents. Many of these materials are neither research reports nor are they necessarily peer reviewed, even if they are reports of scientific studies. These documents can be very useful, however, in gathering background material about a topic or issue and suggesting other sources to include in your review of the literature.

An additional Internet resource available on GPO Access is the Government Information Locator Service (GILS), which is a website for finding publicly available federal information resources, including electronic information resources. The website for GILS is http://www.gils.net/overview.html.

Critical Evaluations of the Literature: Critiques by Experts

Increasingly researchers and practitioners alike are faced with the problem of not only staying abreast of what is new but also critically evaluating and integrating the results across multiple studies. Although there are no universal standards for critically evaluating the research literature, different ways of coping with the information explosion have been developed over the past few decades. Four of these strategies are described in this section: (1) review articles, (2) meta-analysis, (3) practice guidelines, and (4) the Cochrane Library.

All four are examples of tertiary source information; however, there are some major differences among them—some are qualitative, and others are quantitative; some are guidelines for practitioners, and others are tools for researchers; some are locally focused, and others are international in scope. What they represent, however, are resources that you can use in your review the literature. Be aware of their existence and consider using them as adjuncts to the usual electronic bibliographic databases.

Review Articles

In general, a review summarizes or synthesizes what is new or currently known about a topic. Some review articles also provide a critical analysis of the research methods and the quality of the research. Reviews can be found in a variety of print and electronic sources. Some peer-reviewed journals that concentrate on original or primary source papers periodically publish a review article, such as the 1995 paper "Alcohol and Mortality: A Review," which was published in the

Journal of Clinical Epidemiology.[3] In many fields there are journals, such as the *Epidemiological Review* or *Systematic Reviews*, that publish only review articles. Finally, there is a series of annual reviews that has been published since 1932. Currently these reviews cover approximately 41 disciplines (see a list of these volumes in Appendix A). Further information about these and future volumes can be found at http://www.annualreviews.org.

Even reviews need to be read critically.[4,5] There is a growing literature on criteria for evaluating the quality of reviews for researchers,[5] practitioners,[4] and science writers.[56] In addition, guidelines have been developed for what constitutes an acceptable review in the health sciences.[7] Some of the most well-known guidelines for systematic reviews include the PRISMA Statement[1] and the IOM Standards, available at this website: http://iom.nationalacademies.org/Reports/2011/Finding-What-Works-in-Health-Care-Standards-for-Systematic-Reviews.aspx. An example of a critical review of the quality of reviews in epidemiology is a paper titled "Quality of Reviews in Epidemiology,"[8] which was published in 1998.

Meta-Analysis

A meta-analysis consists of a critical evaluation of research studies that statistically combines the results of comparable studies or clinical trials on a specific topic. Unlike review articles, which can be qualitative or narrative in form, a meta-analysis is a statistical tool that can be used to synthesize the findings of different studies quantitatively.

Although a standardized strategy for conducting a meta-analysis has not been accepted, researchers agree on the following procedures:

- Study protocol: The analysis must begin with a protocol that states the purpose, methodology, and criteria for selection of studies.
- Selection of studies: Primary source papers of empirically based studies, usually experimental studies, must be used and documented in the publication.
- Statistical analysis: Statistical procedures for combining the results of these studies must be rigorously followed.

There is continuing disagreement about other issues, including the criteria for including and excluding studies with primary source data, whether or not the papers have been published, and whether the data to be analyzed have to be at the aggregate or individual subject level.[9]

Just as there are criteria for a well-done research study and others for evaluating the quality of a review article, there are also guidelines for a well-done meta-analysis. One set of guidelines was published as a series of articles in the *British Medical Journal* in 1997 and 1998; additional articles are expected to be published in the future.[10–15]

Clinical Practice Guidelines

Clinical practice guidelines were defined in 1992 by the Institute of Medicine (IOM) as "systematically developed statements to assist practitioner and patient decisions about appropriate health care for specific clinical circumstances."[16] Further information is available at the National Guideline Clearinghouse (http:// www.guideline.gov), which is a collection of evidence-based clinical practice guidelines and related documents. The clearinghouse is maintained by AHRQ, which is part of the U.S. Department of Health and Human Services.

Cochrane Library

The Cochrane Library is an electronic library of systematic reviews of health-related research findings produced by the Cochrane Collaboration (http://www .cochrane.org). Although described initially in Chapter 1, this summary in Chapter 3 provides greater detail about the Cochrane Library. A standard protocol is used for all Cochrane reviews. For more information, go to the home page, click the tab, "Cochrane Reviews," read the first paragraph, and click on the highlighted keywords.

The Cochrane Library is rapidly evolving and may eventually become one of the primary international sources of information about the effectiveness of healthcare interventions. This is an important resource for anyone interested in the synthesis of findings about healthcare interventions across multiple research studies. Cochrane reviews, first released in April 1996, are updated on a quarterly basis and are available by institutional subscription, pay per view, or CD-ROM through Wiley InterScience. Many university libraries have an institutional subscription to the Cochrane Library; check with the reference librarian. The abstracts of the reviews are freely available online. Currently the Cochrane Library consists of seven databases based on information at their website: http:// community-archive.cochrane.org/editorial-and-publishing-policy-resource /overview-cochrane-library-and-related-content. At that website, see "Overview of the Cochrane Library and related content."

1. Cochrane Database of Systematic Reviews (CDSR): CDSR is a collection of systematic reviews of the effects of experimental studies of health care. Each review is prepared by one of the voluntary Cochrane collaborative review groups using preapproved protocols for research synthesis, as

specified in the Cochrane review methodology database. The reviews are updated and amended as new evidence becomes available. The CDSR is the primary output of the collaborative. Examples of some of the reviews include the following, as described by the Canadian members of the Cochrane Collaborative based at McMaster University:

- How stroke can be prevented and treated
- Which drugs are effective in the treatment of malaria, tuberculosis, and other infectious diseases
- Which strategies are effective in preventing brain and spinal cord injuries and their consequences

2. Database of Abstracts of Reviews of Effects: This database contains abstracts of other systematic reviews based on explicit criteria and abstracts from health technology agencies from around the world.

3. Cochrane Central Register of Controlled Trials: This is a bibliographic database of randomized clinical trials or experimental studies of healthcare interventions that include trials described in conference proceedings and other sources not usually available in peer-reviewed journals.

4. Cochrane Methodology Reviews: This database includes publications in journals and books about the science of reviewing research. Also included is a handbook of how to conduct a systematic review and a glossary of terms. The database describes how to contact the Cochrane Library and information about collaborative review groups.

5. Cochrane Methodology Register: This is a bibliography of publications about research methods used in controlled trials from journal articles, books, and conference proceedings. The records include the title of the article, where it was published (bibliographic details), and in some cases a summary of the article, but not the full text.

6. Health Technology Assessment Database: This database contains information on healthcare technology assessments, including prevention and rehabilitation, vaccines, pharmaceuticals and devices, medical and surgical procedures, and the systems within which health is protected and maintained. The database includes descriptions of ongoing projects and completed publications from health technology assessment organizations.

7. NHS Economic Evaluation Database: This database contains abstracts of articles describing economic evaluations of healthcare interventions, including the following:

- Cost–benefit analysis, which measures both costs and benefits in monetary values and calculates net monetary gains or losses (presented as a cost–benefit ratio)

- Cost-effectiveness analysis, which compares interventions with a common outcome (such as blood pressure level) to discover which produces the maximum outcome for the same input of resources in a given population
- Cost-utility analysis, which measures the benefits of alternative treatments or types of care by using clearly defined utility measures (such as quality-adjusted life years)

Using Tertiary Source Materials

In reading an article that reviews other scientific papers or studies, results of a meta-analysis, practice guidelines, material from the Cochrane Library, or systematic reviews that use the guidelines, such as the PRISMA Statement[1] or the IOM Standards for Systematic Reviews, pay special attention to the list of papers in the references section. These references may be useful as you search for primary source articles.

Given the effort and expertise that goes into creating many of these tertiary source materials, you may now be wondering why you should do your own review of the literature. Why not simply use the excellent output of others on the topic of your choice? The answer is threefold:

1. The purpose of your review of the literature may not be exactly what has been included in these tertiary source materials.
2. A secondary or tertiary source document will inevitably contain a bias that you may or may not recognize or agree with. (So far as that goes, your literature review of primary source materials is also likely to contain a selection bias.) The advantage of doing your own review is that of experience—you know what the researchers said they did and how you interpreted their methods and results. You do not have that level of understanding if you read someone else's synthesis or review of the same documents.
3. Finally, you will not truly own the literature until you have examined the primary source documents yourself. This is especially important for future research. On the other hand, if your goal is to gain a better understanding about what interventions or treatments are effective, then using one or more of the tertiary source documents may be an important section to add to your literature review.

Each of the four examples of tertiary source information has strengths and weaknesses. Reviews can vary in thoroughness and quality. There are no universal standards for review articles, as has been pointed out by others in the field.

The same concern applies to a meta-analysis. A statistical methodology does not automatically confer objectivity. How the studies were initially selected, the quality of those original studies, and the appropriateness of the meta-analytic techniques are important considerations. Practice guidelines were developed for practitioners, and the quality of the research and ways in which the studies were combined to arrive at the guidelines may vary. Finally, the emphasis in the systematic reviews by the Cochrane Collaborative has usually been on randomized trials. There is a vast amount of useful information from research studies that do not use that methodological design, and those studies are not emphasized in the Cochrane Library. In summary, you should seriously consider using tertiary source documents, but only as an adjunct to primary and secondary source materials.

The Web: Beware of Readily Available Resources

The World Wide Web (www), which is currently the most popular system for accessing the Internet, offers expanding opportunities for reviewers of the literature. One of the first places to explore is the NLM at http://www.nlm.nih.gov. The NLM, which is part of the NIH, developed and maintains MEDLINE and other health-related databases. Both of these sites—NLM and NIH—can also be found by typing their initials in most search engines.

Other sites to explore include professional associations that publish journals, for example, the American Medical Association, which publishes *JAMA*, or the American Sociological Society, which publishes the *Journal of Health and Social Behavior*. Alternatively, you could search for the names of specific journals, such as the *American Journal of Public Health* or *Science*. Appendix A includes a list of some of the more well-known scientific associations and their websites.

Nonfederal Web-Based Citation Indexes

Web-based citation indexes that are not part of the federal government have emerged since approximately 2004. These newcomers fall into two broad categories: those that are free and those that require an institutional or individual subscription.

Examples of the freely accessible indexes include Google Scholar (by the Google search engine), CiteSeer^X (by academics and researchers with a focus on computer and information science), and GetCITED (an online, member-controlled database of academic publications and citations of journal articles and book chapters).

Other citation indexes require a subscription and are often available through libraries, especially university-based libraries. Examples include Scopus (by Elsevier, the publisher) and Thomson ISI's Web of Science, which includes the Science Citation Index (described in the next section). Check with the librarian at your university or public library to see if the library has a subscription to one of these indexes and determine whether or not you can gain free access to them.

In reviewing the literature, the logical question to ask is, Should I use one of these other non-NLM indexes instead of (or in addition to) one of the other more well-established indexes such as MEDLINE (or PubMed)? The answer is still in debate. You might explore one of these, such as Google Scholar, to see for yourself how the results of a limited search compare to those of the same search through PubMed.

Citation Index: A Useful Tool When You Know What You Want

After you are well into the process of locating specific journals and doing an initial reading of primary source materials, determine whether there are some individuals who consistently have been associated with the topic of interest. For example, are there key scientists who were the first to do this kind of research or authors whose seminal papers are almost always cited by others in their publications? If so, consider using the Science Citation Index (or its social sciences counterpart, the Social Science Citation Index) to identify other scientific publications in which the researchers list the papers by the key authors. Citation indexes are available in print (and electronic) form in most research libraries; the reference librarian will be able to help you locate and use such indexes.

In one sense these citation indexes work backwards. For example, suppose that two fictitious researchers, Smith and Jones, published the first major study on quality of life of women with breast cancer in 1956 in the fictitious *Journal of American Health*. Their research was so important that most other researchers in the future cited that original paper. Now, years later, you want to identify all studies on this topic that have been reported since the Smith and Jones 1956 paper. Using the Science Citation Index, you look up Smith and Jones, and among their many publications, you locate the 1956 *Journal of American Health* article. Listed under that article will be a list of other studies, from 1956 to the present, that included the Smith and Jones article in the reference lists of their papers. In other words, the Smith and Jones 1956 paper was cited by these other authors. Such a list could be invaluable in a review of the literature because it quickly and efficiently gives you a list of potentially related articles that you can then examine and consider including in your review of the literature.

Others Kinds of Resources: Recent Developments

There are two other sources of literature related to the health sciences that may become useful over time. They are described here not as a recommendation, but more as a suggestion that you keep an eye on them; check them out over the next few years and decide for yourself whether either might be useful to you as you review the scientific literature.

Grey Literature

This source consists of publications such as papers presented at scientific meetings, preliminary reports, technical reports, or government reports or documents. What makes this literature grey is that it is not produced by commercial publishers and is often very difficult to obtain. The term *grey literature* was described in a nongrey journal in 1990.[17] A professional conference meets periodically, and there is an effort in libraries to increase the acquisition and availability of grey literature about public health and health policy.[18] Ask your reference librarian about the grey literature in the health sciences. Further information about grey literature is located at this website: http://www.greylit.org/about.

Wikipedia

Wikipedia is a free encyclopedia written and edited by the public. It was initially made available online in 2001 and includes a broad range of topics that go beyond health-related information. It is not peer reviewed in the traditional sense of scientific journals, but it is a source that is increasingly being used by the public. Wikipedia can be accessed online at http://en.wikipedia.org.

TIPS ON SEARCHING FOR SOURCE DOCUMENTS

Snowball Technique: Developing Ownership of the Literature

Use what is known in the field as the snowball technique to find more references. A snowball gathers snow as it rolls down the hill, and by the same token your goal should be to use references in the papers or books you have read to gather more references. Even if a particular article in a journal is not relevant to the topic under review, some of the references might be. Build a list of references until you begin to see the same references over and over again. In fact, an author's failure to cite an important article in a current publication might suggest that this author did not fully read the literature, which might also make you question the quality of the study. You will know that you are beginning to own the literature when you read a few sentences about a study cited by an author and you immediately think to yourself, "Oh yes, that was the study by Smith and Jones in which they found that . . ." even before you see the reference to Smith and Jones at the end of the description.

Timeliness of the Science: A Comparison of Sources

One consideration in reviewing the literature is whether or not to include papers that do not appear to be current with what has already known. Unfortunately, by the time a scientific paper is published in a peer-reviewed journal, the results are already out of date in some fields. Probably the most current knowledge about a topic can be found in papers presented at scientific meetings—but this applies only to the day or week they are presented. The disadvantage of presentations at scientific meetings is that they usually have not been subjected to the rigorous review process required of papers published in peer-reviewed journals. Materials made available on the Internet might also be very recent, but they are probably even more suspect if they have not gone through the peer-review process. The exception might be online, full-text papers in peer-reviewed journals such as PLOS (https://www.plos.org). In general, the most recently published studies are papers in scientific journals, followed by those described in the annual reviews, followed, finally, by books.

If you restrict the review to scientific, peer-reviewed, published papers, then how recent is recent? The time from completion of a study (or the end of the study period, because it is not always clear when the study actually ended) to publication varies from study to study and field to field. Try to get a sense of a relative definition of recentness for papers in some journals by noting when the papers were submitted or accepted and when they were published. You will need to delve further, however, to discover how much time elapsed between the completion of the study and when the paper was submitted or accepted.

Take, for example, all of the patient-related articles that were original contributions published in the June 1998 issue of *JAMA*. There were 14 such articles, summarized in **Exhibit 3-3**, of which two did not provide information about when the data were collected or when the study period ended. As shown in the last column of Exhibit 3-3, the range of time elapsed between the end of the data collection period (or end of the study) and the publication of these 12 papers was

EXHIBIT 3-3 Time Elapsed Between End of Study and Publication of Final Results in the June 1998 Issue of the *Journal of the American Medical Association (JAMA)*

Study Description	Date of Publication in JAMA	End of Study Period or Completion of Data Collection*	Number of Months Elapsed: End of Study to Publication
Socioeconomic Factors, Health Behaviors, and Mortality[19]	6/3/98	3/1/94	50
Perceived Prognosis and Treatment Preference[20]	6/3/98	1/1/94	52
Cigarette Smoking and Hearing Loss[21]	6/3/98	1995	29
Depressive Symptoms and Physical Decline[22]	6/3/98	1992	65
Death After Hospital Discharge[23]	6/3/98	1994	41
Low Back Pain in Industry[24]	6/10/98	N/A	N/A
Unintentional Cocaine Overdose[25]	6/10/98	12/31/95	29
Culture, Race, and Breast Cancer Stage[26]	6/10/98	N/A	N/A
Pain Management in Elderly Patients with Cancer[27]	6/17/98	1995	17
HIV Incidence among Young Adults[28]	6/17/98	1993	53
Risk Factors in Ischemic Heart Disease[29]	6/24/98	1990	89
Zinc Gluconate Lozenges for the Common Cold[30]	6/24/98	3/97	15
Adjusting Cesarean Delivery Rates[31]	6/24/98	6/95	36
Gastrostomy Placement and Death in Medicare Beneficiaries[32]	6/24/98	12/93	53

*When only the year of data collection was reported, the ending date was set to December of that year, unless otherwise noted in the paper.
N/A = Not Available.

15 to 89 months. Thus, the information in the (then) latest issue of one of the foremost clinical journals in the world was published 3.67 years, on average, after the data were collected. This is a sobering time gap considering how rapidly treatment protocols turn over due to new developments in the scientific or clinical fields.

Research takes time, and good research often takes a lot of time. In thinking about the number of months or years elapsed between the end of a study and publication of the results, perhaps the most important issue to consider is how recent the findings have to be for the information to be meaningful to healthcare providers and beneficial to their patients.

Caroline's Quest: Managing the Search

For her thesis research, Caroline was interested in studying the characteristics of teenage girls who smoke. She was especially interested in exploring whether there was a link between smoking and depression. In order to design her study, Caroline first needed to know what the research literature had shown about both the prevalence of smoking in that age and gender group and what kinds of characteristics had been studied thus far. She knew from her previous reading that race or ethnic origin, socioeconomic status, and rural or urban location were probably important factors, but she was not sure what other kinds of characteristics had been studied.

After talking with Professor Dickerson, Caroline decided to begin by briefly reading pertinent chapters in a few reference books, then concentrating her search for primary source documents by looking in MEDLINE, and next examining some tertiary source documents beginning with the Cochrane Library and the journal *Systematic Reviews*.

At the library, Caroline skimmed the material on the topic of smoking and teenagers in the reference books and made some notes about these reference materials under key sources in the Paper Trail Folder, as shown in **Exhibit 3-4**.

Then Caroline went to see the reference librarian at the library to better understand how to set up and run a PubMed search. The reference librarian walked

---

EXHIBIT 3-4 Key Sources Page in the Paper Trail Folder in Caroline's Master Folder

Centers for Disease Control and Prevention. *Preventing tobacco use among young people: a report of the surgeon general: at a glance.* Atlanta, GA: National Center for Chronic Disease Prevention and Health Program; 1994.

her through how to do a PubMed search, how to record the parameters she used to conduct the search (including date restrictions and inclusions/exclusions, and other specifications). Although Caroline had already taken the PubMed classes at the library, she greatly appreciated the refresher.

Before doing a MEDLINE search herself, Caroline listed some key words and set some initial restrictions for the search. She decided to focus only on American teenagers, with an age range of 13–18 years, if possible. She also wanted to limit her MEDLINE search to papers published in the most recent 10 years. Due to Professor Dickerson's guidance, she was aware that the definitions and terms for her search could be modified as she learned more about her topic.

Caroline wrote this information in the notes document in her Paper Trail Folder in order to have a record of her decisions about the MEDLINE search. Her notes are shown in **Exhibit 3-5**.

Next she turned to the page titled "key words" in the Paper Trail Folder and described the purpose of her literature review and some of the key words that she would use initially. **Exhibit 3-6** is a record of what she wrote.

Caroline was able to access a variety of electronic bibliographic databases, such as MEDLINE, from the computer in her office, rather than go to the library. She

---

EXHIBIT 3-5 Notes Page in the Paper Trail Folder in Caroline's Master Folder

Subject characteristics:
- Teenage—ages 13–18 years
- Smoking—use cigarette smoking only

Prevalence—be sure to get prevalence (rate of people currently smoking divided by total number at risk for smoking). May need to do this on a year-by-year basis. Wonder if I can get this for the entire age period? May want to set up a graph showing prevalence by year for each age.

Limit search to the following:
- The most recent 10 years, at least initially
- Focus only on American teenagers because they might differ from other cultures
- Separate different race/ethnic groups within the United States (e.g., Caucasian, African American, Asian, American Indian—there may be different characteristics associated with smoking within each group)
- Limit search to English-language journals only
- Check review articles, then go to the actual studies

EXHIBIT 3-6 Key Words Page in the Paper Trail Folder in Caroline's
Master Folder

Purpose

What are the characteristics of teenage girls who smoke during the period
1985 to the present in the United States?

Key Words

smoking

cigarettes

teenage girls

prevalence of smoking among teenage girls

---

also had two options for accessing the MEDLINE database. One was through
PubMed, which was free via the Internet, and the other was through the OVID
system, which was available through the biomedical library she used. Caroline
felt fortunate because Professor Dickerson had told her that not all university
libraries provide OVID free of charge to its users. Each access method had
slightly different capabilities, although both provided a gateway to MEDLINE.
She decided to use the PubMed system initially.

Caroline accessed the Internet, and before going to the PubMed website, she
checked the home page of NLM (http://www.nlm.nih.gov) to see whether any new
features had become available. Then she went directly to the PubMed site to begin
her MEDLINE search. The PubMed screen she went to first is shown in **Figure 3-1**.

Using the PubMed search capability, Caroline began her search with the key
word phrase "smoking/epidemiology" and then restricted the search by the age

FIGURE 3-1 PubMed website that Carolyn accessed to use MEDLINE.

PubMed, the National Library of Medicine.

☐ Prevalence of major cardiovascular risk factors and cardiovascular diseases among Hispanic/Latino
1. individuals of diverse backgrounds in the United States.
Daviglus ML, Talavera GA, Avilés-Santa ML, Allison M, Cai J, Criqui MH, Gellman M, Giachello AL,
Gouskova N, Kaplan RC, LaVange L, Penedo F, Perreira K, Pirzada A, Schneiderman N, Wassertheil-
Smoller S, Sorlie PD, Stamler J.
JAMA. 2012 Nov 7;308(17):1775-84. doi: 10.1001/jama.2012.14517.
PMID: 23117778 [PubMed - indexed for MEDLINE]
Related citations

☐ Cigarette smoking topography among alternative school youth: why African American youth smoke
2. less but are at higher long-term risk.
Peters RJ Jr, Kelder SH, Johnson RJ, Prokhorov AV, Meshack A, Jefferson T, Essien EJ.
J Psychoactive Drugs. 2012 Jul-Aug;44(3):252-8.
PMID: 23061325 [PubMed - indexed for MEDLINE]
Related citations

☐ Smoking in top-grossing US movies, 2011.
3. Glantz SA, Iaccopucci A, Titus K, Polansky JR.
Prev Chronic Dis. 2012;9:120170. doi: 10.5888/pcd9.120170.
PMID: 23017248 [PubMed - indexed for MEDLINE]   Free PMC Article
Related citations

☐ Tobacco brand preference among Mexican adolescents.
4. West JH, Hall PC, Page RM, Trinidad DR, Lindsay GB.
Int J Adolesc Med Health. 2011 Nov 29;24(2):143-8. doi: 10.1515/ijamh.2012.021.
PMID: 22909923 [PubMed - indexed for MEDLINE]
Related citations

FIGURE 3-2 Results of Caroline's initial query of the MEDLINE database using "smoking/epidemiology" as the key word phrase.

PubMed, the National Library of Medicine.

and nationality criteria she had previously established. A copy of Caroline's first query, which retrieved 12,132 documents, is shown in **Figure 3-2**.

Caroline applied the search restrictions she had decided on earlier and recorded the results in the Miscellaneous Notes Subfolder of her Paper Trail Folder. Her search resulted in 2,198 references, as shown in **Exhibit 3-7**.

EXHIBIT 3-7 One of the Notes in the Key Words Subfolder in Caroline's Paper Trail Folder

Key words	Number of References
Smoking/epidemiology	12,132
English language	10,646
Human subjects	10,615
Adolescents	3,770
Females	3,179
1966–2006	2,198

☐ Longitudinal trends in race/ethnic disparities in leading health indicators from adolescence to young
10. adulthood.
Harris KM, Gordon-Larsen P, Chantala K, Udry JR.
Arch Pediatr Adolesc Med. 2006 Jan;160(1):74-81.
PMID: 16389215 [PubMed - indexed for MEDLINE]
Related citations

FIGURE 3-3 Example of a reference from MEDLINE.

PubMed, the National Library of Medicine.

Next, Caroline rapidly scanned the titles and abstracts of each of the 2,198 citations until she found a title relating to adolescents and smoking: the 2006 Harris et al. citation shown in **Figure 3-3**. She went to PubMed and pulled the Harris et al. paper[33] to read the abstract and checked to see if there were additional papers in the references list of the Harris et al. paper that she should add to her own growing list of documents.

Then she returned to the citations list and clicked on "See Related Articles" to find additional studies on the same topics.

Caroline also explored some of the other electronic bibliographic databases, such as CancerLit and CINAHL. She knew from the reference librarian that it was possible to run the same search in PubMed and CINAHL, for example, using the same criteria for the search and come up with different numbers of documents and different sources. The criteria don't differ, but the wealth of information in one database may be superior in the other database for your topic.

Much of what she had found in MEDLINE was included in those two databases, although there were some differences. Then she downloaded the papers that were available electronically. She moved the digital copies to her Source Documents Subfolder. She knew that if the journals were not available online or in the library, she could talk to the reference librarian about getting a copy of what she needed through interlibrary loan.

Later Caroline returned to the Internet to look for reviews in the Cochrane Collaboration. She reasoned that these tertiary source materials might provide additional references of original research studies. She logged on to the Cochrane Collaboration home page at http://www.cochrane.org and clicked the "Review Abstracts" link on the home page to determine whether any Cochrane reviews had been completed for smoking and found a list of reviews to date.

Caroline decided to examine some other tertiary sources. She was particularly interested in looking at the *Annual Review of Public Health* to see if there was an article on her topic. She reasoned that a current review would give her a list of up-to-date references of original studies that would be useful to examine. She first went to the Annual Reviews website (http://www.annualreviews.org) and then to the site for the *Annual Review of Public Health* (http://www.annualreviews .org/journal/publhealth). She did not find any review articles that were specific to her topic; therefore, she decided to concentrate on reading the papers she had downloaded to decide which of those should be included in her review. Then she would use the references from those papers to help her identify additional studies using the snowball technique. Perhaps later she would consider using the Science Citation Index.

What You Should Know or Be Able to Do by the End of This Chapter

1. What is the Paper Trail Folder as used in the Matrix Method? *Your response:* Describe in two or fewer sentences. (Note: If you cannot do this, then review the first part of this chapter.)

2. How do MEDLINE, PubMed, and PMC differ? *Your response:* Describe in one or two sentences.

3. Who is the most important person for you to consult with at the beginning of your Review of the Literature? *Your response:* State the role of the person.

4. Why is it important to record all authors' names in your list of references to source documents in your Paper Trail Folder? *Your response:* Describe in one or two sentences.

5. What is the grey literature? *Your response:* Describe briefly in one or two sentences.

6. Can you do the exact same search in two or more databases online? Will the answers be the same? *Your response:* Describe how this can be done and whether or not the answers from two or more databases will be the same.

REFERENCES

1. Moher D, Liberati A, Tetzlaff T, Altman DG; The PRISMA Group. Preferred reporting items for systematic reviews and meta-analyses: the PRISMA statement. *BMJ.* 2009;339:b2535. doi:http://dx.doi.org/10.1136/bmj.b2535.

2. Garrard J, Harms S, Eberly LE, Matiak A. Variations in product choices of frequently purchased herbs: caveat emptor. *Arch Intern Med.* 2003;163(19):2290-2295.

3. Poikolainen K. Alcohol and mortality: A review. *J Clin Epidemiol.* 1995;48:455-456.

4. Hunt DL, McKibbon KA. Locating and appraising systematic reviews. *Ann Intern Med.* 1997;126:532-538.

5. Weed DL. Methodologic guidelines for review papers. *J Natl Cancer Inst.* 1997;89:6-7.

6. Oxman AD, Guyatt GH, Cook DJ, Jaeschke R, Heddle N, Keller J. An index of scientific quality for health reports in the lay press. *J Clin Epidemiol.* 1993;46:987-1001.

7. Oxman AD. Checklists for review articles. *BMJ.* 1994;309:648-651.

8. Breslow RA, Ross SA, Weed DL. Quality of reviews in epidemiology. *Am J Public Health.* 1998;88:475-477.

9. Fagard RH, Staessen JA, Thijs L. Advantages and disadvantages of the meta-analysis approach. *J Hypertens.* 1996;14(suppl):S9-S13.

10. Egger M, Smith GD. Meta-analysis. Potentials and promise. *BMJ.* 1997;315:1371-1374.

11. Egger M, Smith GD, Phillips AN. Meta-analysis: principles and procedures. *BMJ.* 1997;315:1533-1537.

12. Davey Smith G, Egger M, Phillips AN. Meta-analysis. Beyond the grand mean? *BMJ.* 1997;315:1610-1614.

13. Egger M, Smith GD. Bias in location and selection of studies. *BMJ.* 1998;316:61-66.

14. Egger M, Schneider M, Smith GD. Meta-analysis—spurious precision—meta-analysis of observational studies. *BMJ.* 1998;316:140-144.

15. Davey Smith G, Egger M. Meta-analysis: unresolved issues and future developments. *BMJ.* 1998;316:221-225.

16. Field MJ, Lohr KN. *Guidelines for Clinical Practice: From Development to Use.* Washington, DC: Committee on Clinical Practice Guidelines, Division of Health Care Services, Institute of Medicine; 1992.

17. Alberani V, Pietrangeli P, Mazza A. The use of grey literature in health sciences: a preliminary survey. *Bull Med Libr Assoc.* 1990;78(4):358-363.

18. Gray B. Sources used in health policy research and implications for information retrieval systems. *J Urban Health.* 1998;75(4):842-852.

19. Lantz PM, House JS, Lepkowski JM, Williams DR, Mero RP, Chen J. Socioeconomic factors, health behaviors, and mortality: results from a nationally representative prospective study of US adults. *JAMA.* 1998;279:1703-1708.

20. Weeks JC, Cook EF, O'Day SJ, et al. Relationship between cancer patients' predictions of prognosis and their treatment preferences. *JAMA.* 1998;279:1709-1714.

21. Cruickshanks KJ, Klein R, Klein BE, Wiley TL, Nordahl DM, Tweed TS. Cigarette smoking and hearing loss: the epidemiology of hearing loss study. *JAMA.* 1998;279:1715-1726.

22. Penninx BWJH, Guralnik JM, Ferrucci L, Simonsick EM, Deeg DJH, Wallace RB. Depressive symptoms and physical decline in community-dwelling older persons. *JAMA.* 1998;279:1720-1726.

23. Mullins RJ, Mann NC, Hedges JR, et al. Adequacy of hospital discharge status as a measure of outcome among injured patients. *JAMA.* 1998;279:1227-1231.

24. van Poppel NMN, Koes BW, van der Ploeg T, Smid T, Bouter LM. Lumbar supports and education for the prevention of low back pain in industry: a randomized controlled trial. *JAMA.* 1998;279:1789-1794.

25. Marzuk PM, Tardiff K, Leon AC, et al. Ambient temperature and mortality from unintentional cocaine overdose. *JAMA.* 1998;279:1795-1800.

26. Lannin DR, Mathews HF, Mitchell J, Swanson MS, Swanson FH, Edwards MS. Influence of socioeconomic and cultural factors on racial differences in late-stage presentation of breast cancer. *JAMA*. 1998;279:1801-1807.

27. Bernabei R, Gambassi G, Lapane K, et al. Management of pain in elderly patients with cancer. *JAMA*. 1998;279:1877-1882.

28. Rosenberg PS, Biggar RJ. Trends in HIV incidence among young adults in the United States. *JAMA*. 1998;279:1894-1899.

29. Lamarche B, Tchernof A, Mauriège P, et al. Fasting insulin and apolipoprotein B levels and low-density lipoprotein particle size as risk factors for ischemic heart disease. *JAMA*. 1998;279:1955-1961.

30. Macknin ML, Piedmonte M, Calendine C, Janosky J, Wald E. Zinc gluconate lozenges for treating the common cold in children: a randomized controlled trial. *JAMA*. 1998;279:1962-1967.

31. Aron DC, Harper DL, Shepardson LB, Rosenthal GE. Impact of risk-adjusting cesarean delivery rates when reporting hospital performance. *JAMA*. 1998;279:1968-1972.

32. Grant MD, Rudberg MA, Brody JA. Gastrostomy placement and mortality among hospitalized Medicare beneficiaries. *JAMA*. 1998;279:1973-1976.

33. Harris KM, Gordon-Larsen P, Chantala K, Udry JR. Longitudinal trends in race/ethnic disparities in leading health indicators from adolescence to young adulthood. *Arch Pediatr Adolesc Med*. 2006;160:74-81.

CHAPTER 4

Documents Folder: How to Select and Organize Documents for Review

This chapter is about how to create and use a Documents Folder which has two subfolders: (1) Source Documents Subfolder and (2) PRISMA Flowchart[1] Subfolder. The purpose of the chapter is twofold: (1) how to select, organize, and keep track of all the documents you use in a review of the literature and (2) how to use the PRISMA Flowchart[1] to track the number of source documents as you proceed through your review. This will probably be one of the shortest chapters in the book, but the one that requires the greatest amount of work on your part. The chapter has nine sections:

- Remember to Record the Initial Number of Source Documents
- What to Include in a Source Documents Subfolder
- How to Select Source Documents for Your Review
- How to Organize a Source Documents Subfolder
- How to Remember Where You Put the Documents
- PRISMA Flowchart Subfolder: How to Track the Number of Source Documents from Initiation to Completion of Review
- Caroline's Quest: Assembling and Organizing a Documents Folder
- What You Should Know or Be Able to Do by the End of This Chapter

REMEMBER TO RECORD THE INITIAL NUMBER OF SOURCE DOCUMENTS

From the first time you conduct an electronic review of the literature (when you first run a PubMed search), record in your Paper Trail Folder the total number of source documents identified, including the date the run was made and the criteria for selecting documents in your search strategy. That total number will be your first entry in your copy of the PRISMA Flowchart[1] located in the PRISMA Flowchart Subfolder in this chapter. The number is very important. More about the PRISMA Flowchart[1] will follow later in this chapter, but you need to be alert now as you begin to develop the list of source documents you might be interested in reviewing.

WHAT TO INCLUDE IN A SOURCE DOCUMENTS SUBFOLDER

The Source Documents Subfolder is one of the two subfolders in the Documents Folder; the other one is the PRISMA Flowchart[1] Subfolder. In the Source Documents Subfolder, one copy of each of the papers or source documents is assembled for the literature review. In the years before photocopy machines and before download capabilities were routinely available, you would have written to the author and asked for a reprint of the paper. Most scientific journals offered authors these reprints free or at cost. The practice of requesting a reprint is not as common now as in the past because most journals are available in major research libraries, through interlibrary loan, or more recently as full-text files on the Internet, and users can simply make an electronic copy themselves. The term *reprint* is still with us, however, and occasionally you will hear a collection of journal articles assembled for a review of the literature referred to as a *reprint file*. Thus, the Source Documents Subfolder in the Documents Folder is your reprint file.

You can also think of this subfolder as your database of source documents. Your database will be incomplete, however, because some documents are too large (such as books), unavailable (the journal is not available electronically), or restricted (such as proprietary materials owned by a private company). Nevertheless, maintain a list of all source documents that are important for your review, whether or not a copy is available. Often books can be obtained through interlibrary loan, and a copy of an article in an unavailable journal might be requested through the same source or from the author. Check with your reference librarian.

Proprietary materials present another problem that may not be surmounted, but listing those that appear to be relevant in an appendix in your synthesis will indicate the thoroughness of your search. Bear in mind that proprietary documents are not usually included in the final review of the literature because they are not publically accessible. However, for completeness in your own list of source documents, you should record a citation of such a document in case you eventually find a source that is publicly available. An example might be a formerly classified report that has become declassified.

Advantage of a Source Documents Subfolder

The advantage of maintaining a Source Documents Subfolder is your ability to find your copy of a document when you need it. Even experienced researchers sometimes have trouble locating their copies of source documents. Occasionally these seasoned veterans take the precaution of making multiple copies of the same journal article and spreading the hard copies around in several files to increase the likelihood of finding a copy when they need it. A Source Documents Subfolder solves that problem by providing a reservoir for research articles available for use in a review of the literature. (Caveat emptor: Be sure to back up your computer on a regular basis.)

HOW TO SELECT SOURCE DOCUMENTS FOR YOUR REVIEW

Selecting which documents will be included in the Source Documents Subfolder as possible candidates for your literature review is your next task. Reviewing the abstract, skimming the document, and downloading it as a PDF or scanning the document are the steps for selecting documents.

Review the Abstract

If the document is an original research article, quickly read the abstract to see whether it is relevant to your topic. This strategy is most efficient if the abstract is available online in a database such as MEDLINE or PubMed. Unfortunately, not all papers have an abstract, nor do the electronic bibliographic databases, such as MEDLINE, provide abstracts for some kinds of documents. For example, editorials usually do not include an abstract, yet such a document may include an important issue or a significant reference. Furthermore, some journals do not require an abstract for any of the papers. For documents with those limitations, go to the actual journal or source to determine whether they should be considered for your literature review.

You could also read an abstract of a paper that hasn't reached publication yet, download the preliminary copy as a PDF. Insert that abstract into your Source Documents Subfolder with the current year as publication date, and let it be a placeholder until the actual paper (with a more accurate year of publication) becomes available on PubMed.

Skim the Document

If either the title of the article or the abstract appears to be relevant to your topic or the study has been mentioned in a secondary or tertiary source document, the next step is to examine briefly the full text of the original article. It is more efficient if you can find the article as a full-text, online document (i.e., reprinted in its entirety in electronic form). Sometimes you will not be so fortunate, nor should you limit your search to only those articles available electronically because that could create a form of selection bias.

After you have access to the article, skim it briefly to determine whether it is relevant to your topic. Look not only at the abstract, but also the entire article, including the authors' statement of the purpose, methods section, and results. Consider the possibility that although the topic of a paper may be too specific for your review, the methods or the conclusions might have some relevance to a discussion in your final synthesis of the literature. If that is the case, download the article to your computer and store it in the Source Documents Subfolder; this is discussed further in the next section.

This article selection process alone is just the beginning; it is not sufficient for a review of the literature. Specifically, this stage involves only making a decision about whether or not to store a copy of the source document.

Download a Copy of the Document

Download electronic copies of relevant articles. If you have selected too many documents, create a continuum for yourself from clearly essential to maybe relevant to remotely interesting, and download from the top of the continuum downward until you run out of resources, such as space or time. This means, however, that you may have to return to the source at an inconvenient time to reexamine one or more of the discarded articles. Make sure you place the URL where these papers are located in your Paper Trail Folder or as a PDF in a Word document with notes about the paper used as place holders in your Source Documents Subfolder. Again, use the current year as the initial part of the title and your identifier about the study.

If you want to include a document that is not in an electronic form, you need to talk to a reference librarian about obtaining permission to make one copy for your use. (Usually this is permitted.) It is important to abide by copyright rules in making such a copy. When a copy is available, you can scan it and store it in your Source Documents Subfolder.

HOW TO ORGANIZE A SOURCE DOCUMENTS SUBFOLDER

Just having a copy of a source document in the Source Documents Subfolder does not guarantee that you will be able to find it efficiently the next time you need it. To bring order to the Source Documents Subfolder, organize the research articles chronologically by year of publication. Then store the subfolder in the Documents Folder (in the Master Folder) in EndNote. EndNote is very useful in case you switch from one computer to another.

As you can see in **Exhibit 4-1**, each of the documents in the Source Documents Subfolder was downloaded as a PDF file. I always use the publication year of the paper as the first piece of information in the title of each PDF and provide my own brief description of the paper, sometimes with name of authors, or other information. I don't necessarily use all of these source documents in the Review

---

EXHIBIT 4-1 Source Documents Subfolder Stored in My Documents Folder Located in EndNote

- 📄 2004 Qual res methds…ials in systematic reviews
- 📄 2009 checklist (N=27 items) of original PRISMA
- 📄 2009 Initial PRISMA sta…t Moher et al | The BMJ
- 📄 2009 PRISMA Explanation & Elaboration.pdf
- 📄 2009 PRISMA Statement Liberati et al (BMJ)
- 📄 2009 The PRISMA state…d elaboration | The BMJ
- 📄 2013 Yoga & Low back pain Paper pdf
- 📄 2013 Yoga for low back…tract - PubMed Abstract
- 📄 2015 (PRISMA-P) 2015 | The BMJ
- 📄 2015 Description of PRISMA-P by developers
- 📄 2015 Nursing review of aggression to nurses
- 📄 2015 PRISMA extensio…twork Meta-analyses.pdf
- 📄 2015 PRISMA_IPD (JAMA).pdf
- 📄 2015 Yoghurt & weight mgt Systematic Rreview
- 📄 2016 Choi & De Gagne paper
- 📄 PLOS Medicine Living Systematic Reviews

Matrix, but it is nice to have them handy in case I need to consider them as I write. This is a useful strategy for me.

The goal of this chronological sequence is twofold: (1) to arrange the source documents in the subfolder for use in the next step, which involves constructing the Review Matrix, and (2) to provide a quick index for efficiently finding a particular source document at a later time. The chronological order is automatic; I don't have to insert a paper published in 2003 before 2004—it is done automatically. When you have reached the point of diminishing returns by apparently exhausting all the source documents that can be added, you are ready to advance to the next step, that of constructing the Review Matrix. Bear in mind, however, that you probably will find more source materials to add to the Source Documents Subfolder while you construct the Review Matrix and even later when you write a synthesis of the literature.

HOW TO REMEMBER WHERE YOU PUT THE DOCUMENTS

Losing track of where you stored your reprints is an occupational hazard. Researchers, policy analysts, science writers, and other professionals in the health sciences who systematically and critically review the literature on multiple subjects face this problem. Regardless of the scope of the tasks or the setting, practically everyone experiences this problem—how to find his or her materials, even when the information is stored appropriately in a Source Documents Subfolder. Some kind of tracking or indexing system is needed. A simple tracking system is described, based only on the year of publication and a few key words in the title. It will suffice to get you started.

More Than One Master Folder

Eventually, you probably will have multiple Master Folders in your library. If so, give them different labels. For example, one might be the Diabetes Master Folder, and another might be the Maternal and Child Health Master Folder, which were created when you conducted two separate reviews of the literature. If you *consistently* use the term *Master Folder*, it is easier for you to use those as key words in a search for all the Master Folders on your desktop. Consistency in naming pays off!

Likewise, when you create each of the four folders that make up the Master Folder, such as a Documents Folder within each of those master folders, then give it the same label as the Master Folder, for example, Diabetes Documents Folder or Maternal and Child Health Documents Folder. Labeling the folders with short names is best; this saves a lot of keyboarding.

The key to accessing your own store of information quickly and efficiently is to create a tracking system. Suppose that you have added new source documents to one of the Documents Folders over the past several years. How do you remember what is there? You need a system that lists the contents of each Master Folder and its four main folders (i.e., Paper Trail Folder, Documents Folder, Review Matrix Folder, and Synthesis Folder).

A more sophisticated strategy for indexing the contents of an expanding number of Master Folders is the Matrix Indexing System, described in Chapter 8 of this book. You aren't there yet if this is your first review of the literature. The simpler approach is the tracking system described above using year of publication as the first part in the title of the source document. Whichever system you use, the benefits accrue only if you keep the list up to date.

PRISMA FLOWCHART SUBFOLDER: HOW TO TRACK THE NUMBER OF SOURCE DOCUMENTS FROM INITIATION TO COMPLETION OF REVIEW

The PRISMA Flowchart Subfolder is the second of the two subfolders in the Documents Folder. This is where you will record the number of documents you identify as you progress through each stage of the review of the literature. The PRISMA Flowchart[1] was described initially in Chapter 1 of this book, but now it takes on a more concrete form. Here is what you must do:

After creating the PRISMA Flowchart Subfolder, store a copy of the PRISMA Flowchart,[1] which you will modify as you go along from Chapters 3 through 6. **Exhibit 4-2** is a copy of the original PRISMA Flowchart[1] as described in the 2009 paper about the PRISMA Statement.[1]

There are some changes you need to make to this generic version of the PRISMA Flowchart[1] at the very beginning. First, you can download this yourself from the Moher et al. article.[1] Go to the BMJ website, call up the article, download the flowchart, insert the flowchart to a Word document, and make the following changes:

1. Type your title above the flowchart (e.g., Exhibit 4-2. PRISMA Flowchart of Number of Documents in the Literature Review). Cite the reference to the Moher et al. paper here.[1]

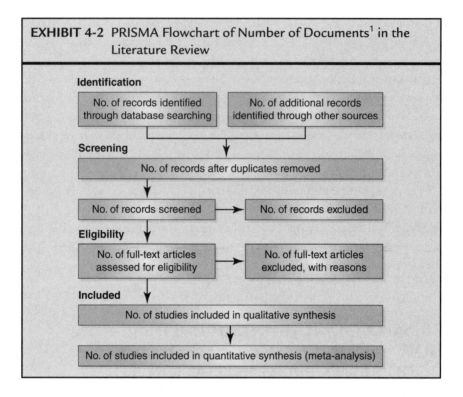

EXHIBIT 4-2 PRISMA Flowchart of Number of Documents[1] in the Literature Review

Identification

No. of records identified through database searching

No. of additional records identified through other sources

Screening

No. of records after duplicates removed

No. of records screened → No. of records excluded

Eligibility

No. of full-text articles assessed for eligibility → No. of full-text articles excluded, with reasons

Included

No. of studies included in qualitative synthesis

No. of studies included in quantitative synthesis (meta-analysis)

2. Add the number of your source documents, wherever the PRISMA authors put **"No"** for number. You will not have the final numbers until you are through with writing your synthesis, but recording the ones you do have, such as total number of documents found initially and those rejected after you applied your search criteria, will be possible.

3. Add categories of reasons why records were removed under **Screening**, and again under **Eligibility** together with the number of documents within each category.

4. Finally, remove the bottom line, **No of studies included in quantitative synthesis (meta-analysis)**. At this stage in your career, you are not doing a meta-analysis. This option is also beyond the scope of this book.

Modify this flowchart by adding the number of source documents at each stage of your review of the literature as you progress through the remaining Matrix Method chapters in this book. You are strongly urged to make a copy of the PRISMA Flowchart[1] with the current date, every time you add or change a number. Keep these copies in your PRISMA Flowchart Subfolder. You will eventually be including your completed PRISMA Flowchart[1] in your final paper, as described in Chapter 6 of this book.

This chapter has a lot in it. You have downloaded PDFs of the source documents you might be interested in reviewing, organized them in the Source Documents Subfolder (preferably saved in your EndNote app) by year of publication with a simple title of your choice. This organization will be useful in the next chapter when you read and abstract each study.

In this chapter, you have also downloaded, modified, and begun to fill in your numbers in the PRISMA Flowchart[1] that will eventually be part of your final synthesis. Your copies of the PRISMA Flowchart[1] are stored in the PRISMA Flowchart Subfolder in the Documents Folder.

Caroline's Quest: Assembling and Organizing a Documents Folder

Caroline's next task was to choose which of the 15 research articles she would abstract in the review matrix. First she sorted the papers by year of publication and began with the oldest paper, published in 1992. She read the abstract and skimmed the entire paper, making a few notes about questions she would return to later when she abstracted the final set of papers. At this point Caroline was not doing any abstracting. In fact, she had not even decided which column topics she would use as the basis for abstracting the studies. As she read, however, she made notes of potential topics for the review matrix. Of the 15 papers she scanned, Caroline chose nine of the studies as possible candidates for abstracting in the review matrix on characteristics of adolescent girls who smoke.

"Well, that step was easy," Caroline commented to Professor Dickerson at their weekly meeting. She showed him the Master Folder on her laptop with her notes in the Paper Trail Folder and the copies of the nine articles in the Source Documents Subfolder in the Documents Folder.

"What happened to the six papers you decided not to include?" Professor Dickerson asked.

Caroline described how she chose only the most relevant ones.

Professor Dickerson understood her logic, but he cautioned, "You might want to leave the other six papers you found in your Source Documents Subfolder even if you don't use them. Why don't you create another subfolder for those six articles, perhaps titled 'Papers Not Included Source Documents Subfolder' in your Documents Folder?"

He paused at her quizzical look and added, "I've found that sometimes a study is referred to by an author and I wonder if I shouldn't consider it. If I have deleted it from my Source Documents Subfolder, then I have to go find it again. But if I just leave it in that subfolder or create another subfolder, then

I know I've read the abstract and realized it wasn't useful. Since you've got a lot of storage space, think about the practice of including and organizing every paper you download."

Caroline made a note of this advice.

Professor Dickerson continued, "Caroline, you need to track the number of source documents you identified, considered, and eventually used or not in your literature review. It's easier to do this as you go along, rather than at the end of your literature review. You also need to make a final run of your search strategy for documents, using the set of instructions you have stored in your Paper Trail Folder. If new studies have been added in this final run, then consider them as you have the others: should you exclude them at different stages of your review, if not, then critically abstract them just as you did the others.

After that, consider the numbers you put in your copy of the PRISMA Flow-chart[1] as final and clearly define the inclusion/exclusion criteria for each stage of the flowchart. You are not responsible for any papers published after that final date, even if one of them is groundbreaking. However, when you defend your thesis, you should describe the groundbreaking paper briefly just to show how VERY up to date you are in this review."

Caroline nodded. This she understood.

"Now, filing reprints is easy," Professor Dickerson continued. "But your job isn't done yet. You need to constantly be alert for more studies as you read each of these articles. If you find that there are some authors who are referenced frequently, look them up in Science Citation Index to see whether you can find additional studies that also cited them." He grinned. "Use the snowball technique to find more studies, add them to the Source Documents Subfolder and include them in your review. Remember, this stage comes well before you make a final run for your PRISMA Flowchart,"[1] he advised.

"What if I haven't found all the right studies?" Caroline looked concerned. "I could be missing something that is a classic in the field and not even know it. Reviewing the literature seems like such a hit or miss kind of thing, even with the Matrix Method."

Professor Dickerson nodded, "I agree. You must constantly be looking for more studies. Abstracting the ones you have will probably help. You want to reach the point where you have the sense that you know who the researchers are and what research questions they have studied. In other words, you need to begin to own the literature."

"Okay, I understand how to use the source documents. But what if I have the opposite problem? What if all the documents I want to use have been gathered together already, say, in a special report online? Do I have to make a copy of each one and put them in a Source Documents Subfolder to do a review of the literature?" Caroline was thinking about the effort it would take to find and download each of the papers—all in different journals, no doubt.

"No." Professor Dickerson responded. "If the documents are available elsewhere and are convenient to use, you do not have to download a copy. The Source Documents Subfolder is meant to be a convenience for you and an organized way of maintaining a reprints file." He thought a minute and then continued, "Frankly, Caroline, I don't know of many situations in which all of the documents for a literature review have already been assembled in one place. You also need to think about what to do with the articles themselves. One of the advantages of having a copy of the original article is being able to mark it up as you read it. If possible, turn on track changes in your word processor and insert comments. You can highlight certain key parts or write questions to yourself on a sticky note or create another blank document and write your questions and answers there. If you are working from an original in another database, you probably can't mark it up."

He paused to let Caroline think about the pros and cons of downloading copies of the documents for review, and then he continued, "Your task next week will be to make decisions about which column topics to use in your review matrix."

What You Should Know or Be Able to Do by the End of This Chapter

Your knowledge about what you should know or be able to do lies in your ability to complete the instructions in this section. Specifically, you should do the following:

1. Organize your Documents Folder. Create two major subfolders: Source Documents and PRISMA Flowchart.[1] Download each of the source documents you might want to abstract (not all 1,000 that you identified initially, but probably more than the 21 you will eventually use) and store them in chronological order in the Source Documents Subfolder.

2. Label each PDF file of each document with the year of publication and a brief title. This is your reprint file.

3. In the next step, as you reject a source document, perhaps label it, "Reject-cite reason," in the title and store it in a separate subfolder

(i.e., Papers Not Included Subfolder, in your Documents Folder. This helps to complete the final numbers in the PRISMA Flowchart.[1]

4. Download the PRISMA Flowchart.[1] Modify it as instructed, and start putting in your numbers for your literature review. This flowchart won't be complete at this point, but it is easier to do this as you go along.

5. Get all of that accomplished. Now you are ready for the abstracting process as described in the next chapter.

REFERENCE

1. Moher D, Liberati A, Tetzlaff J, Altman DG; The PRISMA Group. Preferred reporting items for systematic reviews and meta-analyses: the PRISMA Statement. *BMJ.* 2009;339:b2535. doi:http://dx.doi.org/10.1136/bmj.b2535.

CHAPTER 5

Review Matrix Folder: How to Abstract the Research Literature

This chapter focuses only on the Review Matrix. There is further information about the PRISMA Flowchart[1] in the next chapter as you write your synthesis review. In this chapter, I describe how to organize a Review Matrix Folder, how to choose column topics, select which documents to include, and analyze each of the source documents based on these topics. The sections of this chapter are as follows:

- What Is a Review Matrix?
- How to Organize a Review Matrix Folder
- How to Construct a Review Matrix: Rule of Rows
- How to Choose Column Topics for a Review Matrix
- How to Select and Organize Documents in a Review Matrix
- How to Analyze Documents in a Review Matrix
- Fringe Benefits of the Abstracting Process
- Caroline's Quest: Constructing and Using a Review Matrix
- What You Should Know or Be Able to Do by the End of This Chapter

WHAT IS A REVIEW MATRIX?

A matrix is a rectangle with rows and columns, like a spreadsheet. In a Review Matrix, the rows are for documents, such as journal articles, and the columns are for the topics you will use to abstract each of those documents. A summary of an article in a Review Matrix describes only the most pertinent information

Table 5-1 Generic Review Matrix

Topic 1	Topic 2	Topic 3	Topic 4
Example: Author, Title, Journal	*Example: Year*	*Example: Purpose*	*Example: Type of Study Design*
Journal article 1	1995	Drug treatment for epilepsy	Experimental study
Journal article 2	1997	Drug treatment for depression	Case-control study

about the topic. **Table 5-1** shows a generic example in which the first two rows are journal articles and the columns are the first four topics of the Review Matrix.

Here is an example. Suppose you were interested in the (fictitious) 1987 article, "The Cure for the Common Cold," by the fictitious Professor Brown. In your Review Matrix, you would include his paper in the first row, and the topics to be used in describing that paper would be listed across the top of the Review Matrix. Professor Brown's archrival, Professor White, published a similar paper in 1989, which you also described. **Table 5-2** illustrates how those two papers would look in the first part of a Review Matrix.

Thus, a Review Matrix is a rectangular arrangement, or a matrix, in which the rows always have the journal articles or papers listed down the left side, and the topics or issues that you are going to use to abstract each article are the column headings, always listed across the top of the table.

Advantages of a Review Matrix

The reason for using the Matrix Method is to create order out of chaos. In a review of the literature, the chaos that you must deal with is too much information spread across too many journal articles or other source documents with too

Table 5-2 Review Matrix for Literature on Cure for the Common Cold

Author, Title, Journal	Year	Purpose	Methodological Design
Brown, CJ. Cure for the common cold. *Journal of Scientific Wonder.*	1987	Compare drug X with a placebo for cold cure	Randomized clinical study
White, RM. A better cure for the common cold. *Journal of Better Science.*	1989	Compare drug Y with drug X for superior cold cure	Randomized clinical trial

many details to remember. The order you are going to impose is organizing this information so you can think about it and use it efficiently. The Review Matrix provides a standard structure for creating order. Constructing a Review Matrix is like building a house. You will still need to furnish the house, in this case by reading and analyzing each article and putting that information in each cell, but the Review Matrix provides a place for everything, which allows you to concentrate on the information itself.

HOW TO ORGANIZE A REVIEW MATRIX FOLDER

First you need to organize the Review Matrix Folder. Create three subfolders, Review Matrix-CURRENT, Review Matrix-PREVIOUS, Review Matrix-FINAL, and put them in your Review Matrix Folder.

Set these three subfolders up at the beginning before you put anything in the Review Matrix. During each working session, save your Review Matrix-CURRENT Subfolder often as you fill in the column topics for each source document. At the end of the session save it again and leave it in the Review Matrix-CURRENT Subfolder. There should be only one copy of your Review Matrix in the Review Matrix-CURRENT Subfolder at any one time. Here are examples of how to do this:

1. **Review Matrix-CURRENT Subfolder**

   This subfolder has the most current draft of your Review Matrix. As you work on your Review Matrix, always include the current date with the title and always store it in the Review Matrix-CURRENT Subfolder. Save this file often during your work session. Here is how your label should look:

   2-15-2016 Review Matrix

   File it in the Review Matrix-CURRENT Subfolder. At the beginning of your next working session, open the 2-15-2016 Review Matrix saved from the previous session and create another copy with "save as"; now you have two identical copies. Change the previous date to the current date on one of those copies.

   2-17-2016 Review Matrix

   Now move the older file, 2-15-2016 Review Matrix, to the Review Matrix-PREVIOUS Subfolder.

2. **Review Matrix-PREVIOUS Subfolder**

   Over time, you will build up a number of copies of your Review Matrix in this second subfolder, each organized by date. Be sure to leave the date of the working session on each title so you can determine which is the most recent or perhaps the one you need. Always keep all of your copies of your Review Matrix files in this PREVIOUS Subfolder. You may never know when you will need to go back through these copies in the Review Matrix-PREVIOUS Subfolder to find some information that has somehow disappeared from your current copy.

3. **Review Matrix-FINAL Subfolder**

When you have finalized your Review Matrix, probably when you are writing the synthesis, save the most recent copy in the Review Matrix-CURRENT Subfolder as usual, make a second copy and put it in the Review Matrix-FINAL Subfolder. Here is an example:

4-19-2016 Review Matrix

There should be only one copy of your Review Matrix in the Review Matrix-FINAL Subfolder.

By creating and using these three subfolders, you always will know (1) where to go to find your most current copy of the Review Matrix, (2) provide yourself with insurance for finding the most recent copy of your Review Matrix in the PREVIOUS Subfolder, in case your current copy has become corrupted, and (3) always be able to find your final copy of the Review Matrix at a later date. I speak from experience of having lost a Review Matrix or two before following my own advice!

HOW TO CONSTRUCT A REVIEW MATRIX: RULE OF ROWS

Constructing a Review Matrix as a basis for writing a synthesis of a literature review is a three-step process:

1. **Choosing the column topics:** Set up the Review Matrix on your computer desktop using either the table function in a word processor or a spreadsheet, and decide which column topics to use for this review of the literature.

2. **Organizing the source documents:** After choosing the column topics, select which source documents you want to analyze and organize them chronologically in your Review Matrix. Select these documents from those in the Source Documents Subfolder in the Documents Folder in Chapter 4.

3. **Abstracting the documents:** Now read and abstract each source document under each of the column topics, one at a time, in chronological order, from oldest to most recent. Record your notes under each topic in the cells of the Review Matrix. When preparing a Review Matrix,

remember my "**Rule of Rows**": Abstract each paper one at a time. Finish that paper before going on to the next paper, located in the next row of the Review Matrix.

What follows are the instructions for how to carry out each of these three steps.

HOW TO CHOOSE COLUMN TOPICS FOR A REVIEW MATRIX

What Is a Column Topic?

In a review of the literature, the four most important organizational decisions you will make are (1) stating the purpose of the literature review, (2) defining the search strategy for selecting documents from electronic bibliographic databases or other sources, (3) choosing the column topics, and (4) deciding which source documents to include in the Review Matrix. Column topics in a Review Matrix are the issues or concepts used to abstract each journal article or other source document.

For example, if one of the column topics is "sampling design," then your task in completing a Review Matrix is to identify the type of design used to select subjects for every abstracted study. If the authors did not describe the sampling design, then record its absence by noting that it is not available (NA) or give your best guess, for example, "NA—probably volunteer subjects."

Categories of Column Topics

Rarely will a review of the literature be so comprehensive as to include all of the column topics possible. As you review the scientific literature, consider two broad categories in thinking about the column topics you choose: (1) methodological characteristics of the study and (2) content-specific characteristics, such as the theoretical or conceptual model, the types of results, or the implications for policy or clinical practice.

Most studies published in scientific journals in the health and behavioral sciences literature follow a standard format and include a common set of methodological characteristics describing how the study was designed and analyzed. In choosing column topics, consider some of these methodological characteristics. Examples are shown in Chapter 2 under the Methods Map.

Because these methodological topics will not be sufficient to describe a body of research, be sure to include topics that cover the content of the research. Choose topics based on their relevance to the purpose of your literature review.

First Three Column Topics

Make it a practice to always let the first three columns for each source document in the Review Matrix be the same. Use these three columns to record fundamental information about each source document you abstract:

- Column 1: Author(s), title, name of journal
- Column 2: Year of publication
- Column 3: Purpose of the paper or source document

In the first column, record *all* the names of multiple authors of a paper or book, not just the first three followed by "et al." By including all authors, you will be in a better position to track all the researchers involved in this kind of research. Look for the same researchers as authors of other papers later, even if they are not published together.

Setting aside a column for the year is important because that is the basis on which you will sort and index all source documents and the reprints in the Source Documents Subfolder and in the Review Matrix. The year of publication is the key to finding copies of articles quickly and efficiently.

The third column is used to describe the purpose of the source document—why was the study done, or what was the purpose of the document? State the purpose in your own words. For a research study, try to describe the purpose as a research question. If you (or the authors of the paper) cannot describe the intended purpose in the form of a question, how can you (or they) know whether the question was answered? Describing the purpose may be difficult at times. Some authors do not provide a clear statement of purpose in the introduction section of a paper, and you may have to read the entire paper to determine what they intended to do.

The choice of the rest of the topics is up to you. This is a judgment call that will be based on the purpose of your literature review and your knowledge about the topic. Although there are no rules for generating a list of topics or choosing among them, what follows are some suggestions for a process that may be useful.

Process for Choosing the Remaining Topics

What if you do not know what topics to choose other than the first three? Even if you are doing a literature review to find out something about the latest research in an unfamiliar field, you already know something about the topic. By the time you are ready to choose the column topics for a Review Matrix, you will have consulted reference books about the topic, read numerous abstracts in an electronic bibliographic database or in journals, and skimmed the papers in the

Source Documents Subfolder. The following four-step process in deciding which column topics to use is summarized here:

Step 1: Read a Sample of Papers in the Source Documents Subfolder

Select a sample of source documents that covers the entire time span of articles in your Source Documents Subfolder. Here is an example:

> You have 100 source documents in the Source Documents Subfolder. Randomly select 20% of these from the chronological list (e.g., select the first one, the oldest, and then every 20th one until you have drawn a total of 20 source documents for this sample). Read all the articles or source documents in the sample you selected in chronological order so you can grasp the scope of the research.

This process will begin to give you a sense of how the research issues and methodologies have changed over time. For this second brief reading of a sample of the articles, the purpose is to gain enough of a perspective to choose column topics. Note that some of the documents may not be in electronic form. For example, you may have selected chapters in books or government reports. If possible, make a PDF file copy of the reports. You can create a document in your Source Documents Subfolder consisting of the citation for each of these non electronic materials and then refer to the hard copy when necessary.

Step 2: List Important Issues

As you read this sample of source documents, make a list of the most important issues, both methodological and content specific. For example, if some of the earlier studies used observational designs but later ones used experimental designs, then the type of methodological design might be an important topic. Alternatively, if the area you are reviewing is limited to Medicare recipients, then make a note of this in a "subjects" column of this selection criterion, but do not devote a column to a topic that will be the same for all studies.

Step 3: Select Column Topics

As you are reading a sample of your source documents, create a list of the topics that seem to be the most important from two standpoints: issues in the field and the purpose of your literature review. For example, suppose that you are reviewing the literature on worldwide epidemiology of HIV, and you are especially interested in the rates in South American countries compared to other parts of the world. With regard to content, you might set aside a column for how HIV status was assessed in each study. For purposes of your review, you might include another column for the country in which the subjects resided. Better yet, you could assign a number, such as "1" to source documents about South American studies and "2" for all other countries. A column with quantitative codes can be sorted in a Word document with a table option or an Excel spreadsheet.

Step 4: Add Column Topics

After you have begun to abstract the first few source documents, you may need to add other column topics. Additional topics can be added at any time. Sometimes it is not possible to know the full range of topics until you have abstracted all of the documents. (If that happens, then the philosophy of the Review Matrix is working; the abstracting process enabled you to identify an important topic that you had not seen when you began.) Add the missing topic and abstract all the papers again, just on that topic.

A Matter of Thoroughness

At this point, you may be thinking that this amount of detail and effort requires too much commitment on your part, especially when your counterparts have already accomplished their review of the literature in a tenth of the time by simply using a search engine to locate a few studies and then summarizing them.

Whether or not to proceed is fundamentally a decision that only you can make. Think about why you are doing a review of the literature and what the consequences will be of your not doing it thoroughly. If you are trying to understand what is known about a specific subject or if you want to identify what is missing in a body of research, then you must own the literature. Can you take the chance that you have overlooked an important paper? Are you willing to design your own research study without knowing whether another researcher has already addressed that very question? How thorough is thorough enough?

This also raises the questions of (a) how many papers or source documents is enough, and (b) what is a specific number to aim for? The answer to each of those question is (a) I don't know, but you will, and (b) no, there is no specific number. As you begin to read the source documents, ask yourself these questions:

- What is the time frame of this review? Should I examine research over the past 5 or 10 years? Was there a seminal event, such as the mapping of the human genome, that marked a clear turning point in this research? Should I use that as the beginning of this time frame? You could go back 10 years before this event and therefore increase the number of papers you select, but that might not be logical based on the purpose of your review.
- How specifically should the subject of this review be defined? For example, if the review is of outcomes of total knee replacement surgery, was there

a specific type of replacement part that you are interested in? If so, that becomes part of the definition you are using. Perhaps there have only been seven papers published about this replacement part. You may want to broaden your definition. Alternatively, seven could be the total number of papers you include, and that number would be sufficient.

There is no thoroughness index that will tell you when you have done enough. Your only guide to determining thoroughness is your own sense of knowing the literature well enough to own it. The Matrix Method is one way of approaching that type of ownership, but it is not a guarantee of thoroughness. If you decide to continue, then the next step is to select the source documents to include in your Review Matrix. Read each source document thoroughly and abstract it based on the column topics. Then read and abstract the next source document until all have been examined.

HOW TO SELECT AND ORGANIZE DOCUMENTS IN A REVIEW MATRIX

In constructing the Review Matrix, you will arrange all source documents from the oldest to the most recent by year of publication, just as you did the larger set of documents in the Source Documents Subfolder. Later as you analyze these documents, you may want to re-sort a copy of the Review Matrix by study characteristics. For example, sort by methodological design (e.g., experimental, quasi-experimental, pre-experimental, other), or by study outcomes (e.g., those that support, refute, or cannot determine a positive outcome). Play around with the Review Matrix at this point to help you think about different ways of viewing the studies. But be sure to make a copy of the original Review Matrix before you start this playful bit of inquiry.

Most of the source documents that you will abstract in the Review Matrix will be research papers and other journal articles or book chapters, and these were stored in chronological order as PDFs and saved in the Source Documents Subfolder (in Chapter 4). At this point, you will transfer only the source documents you have selected for writing your synthesis. As you get into the process of analyzing the documents in the next chapter and writing a synthesis, you may find it necessary to include source documents. Put their PDFs in the Source Documents Subfolder in Chapter 4, insert them in your Review Matrix, and analyze each by the column topics.

HOW TO ANALYZE DOCUMENTS IN A REVIEW MATRIX

Taking Notes

What do you actually do when you analyze an article? At the simplest level, you summarize the topic in the area, or cell, where the row and column meet in the Review Matrix. By now you have read each article up to two times, first to decide whether to download it to the Source Documents Subfolder and second to make a decision about which column topics to use based on a sample of these documents. Now comes the third and most intensive reading in which you will critically analyze the source documents. You will abstract each document on the basis of the column topics, and in the process you will fill in the cells of the Review Matrix.

Essential Tools: Calculator, Highlighter, and Sticky Notes

Never read an empirical paper without a calculator. Check the numbers and the percentages. Do the number of subjects in the tables of results add up to the number the researchers said they enrolled at the beginning of the study? All of this will help you understand what the authors did in conducting their study. Two other important tools to have at hand when critically reading a research paper are the highlighter tool in your word processor or spreadsheet for marking important sections of the paper and a sticky note or comment tool in your software for writing notes and questions on the paper itself.

Re-create the Study in Your Mind

Be forewarned that simply recording information in the Review Matrix without reconstructing the study in your own mind does not constitute a critical review of the literature. In order to read a scientific paper thoroughly, you must essentially re-create the study by retracing the authors' steps. Begin by asking yourself questions such as what was their purpose, how did they go about doing the study, what were their results, and what was their logic in their interpretation of their findings? In the process of understanding what the authors did, determine whether you agree scientifically with their purpose, methods, results, and interpretations. That is the critical part of critically reviewing the literature.

In one sense, each scientific paper is a story—a true story—and you have to re-create that story accurately in your own words to understand the paper fully. Make electronic notes in the margins of the paper as you read it. You might use the "Track Changes" feature in your word processor for this purpose. Highlight words that you do not understand or terms that the authors did not define and look them up. Highlight important parts of the paper, such as the purpose or key results, and draw diagrams of the time relationships. For example, when was the pretest administered? How much later was the intervention? How long did the intervention last, and how long after that was the posttest? How well did the authors convey the results to the readers? Here you could use the Methods Map from Chapter 2 to diagram each study.

Read the Documents in Chronological Order

The chronological order in which you read the papers is also important. Begin with the oldest paper, based on its publication date, and end with the most recent. The reason for reading in chronological order is that the research of later papers should build on the results of a previous body of work. Perhaps the findings of one paper suggested a new theory for a future study, a new analytical method became available, or an old study was reanalyzed.

Of course the progress that you may see over time depends on the range of papers selected for your review, and there may be gaps in the progression of the science because of papers you overlooked or decided not to analyze. If this appears to be the case, you can always go back and include the missing articles.

Write Notes in the Matrix

In constructing a Review Matrix, your task is to take each article or source material and record notes based on the column topics. The notes in the cells of the Review Matrix have to be concise and very short. Their purpose is to allow you to track the details of a study, not to summarize the entire article.

Occasionally you will have included an article that is a review of other studies or a theoretical paper. In this case you might want to ignore the column topics and make a note in the Review Matrix for that row about the importance of that paper or whether it is a good summary. (Practical tip: In using the table option in a Word document, select that row, go to the Table tab, select Merge Cells, and then write your note for that study across all the cells for that row.)

If you have included several review articles, you might want to create a sub-folder in your Review Matrix just for review articles. This might bring more clarity to your analysis by concentrating on studies that report original empirical research, then analyze the review articles separately.

Other papers may include important points or quotes that you will want to remember without having to search back through all of the documents in the

Review Matrix. Write these more detailed notes in another document or on the computer equivalent of a sticky note and make a note in the matrix where further information was recorded.

An example of the process of reading a research paper in preparation for abstracting it in the Review Matrix is shown in **Exhibit 5-1**.

EXHIBIT 5-1 How to Abstract a Research Paper

Introduction Section

Begin with the introduction section of the paper. Rephrase the authors' purpose in your own words. Put it in the form of a research question. If the authors have not included a purpose—some do not—then state what you think their question is and make a note that they did not state the purpose.

Methods Section

Read and reread each part of the methods section of the paper until you have a clear idea of what the authors did. Sometimes authors (or editors) leave out important information. If so, describe what you think they did—but make a note that this was your opinion. In order to really understand the study, you need to re-create what the authors did in carrying it out. In other words, describe for yourself the procedures they used.

Now look at the numbers in the subsection about subjects and how they were selected for the study. Begin with the number of subjects—is it possible to trace how many were in the sample at the beginning of the study and how many subjects were lost as the study progressed? Subjects get lost for a variety of reasons; they might have died or moved away or simply not responded. This is where your calculator comes in. Figure out what the real response rate was; do not depend on the authors' calculations.

The reason this response rate is so important is that researchers run the risk of a sample bias if the characteristics of the sample of subjects who end the study differ from those who began the study. For example, the authors may report that the response rate to a questionnaire was 87% (that is, 87% of the people who were asked to fill out the questionnaire actually did) or that the completion rate for an intervention was 45%. Anything less than 100% raises the possibility of a sample bias, but a rate alone does not indicate sample bias. The authors must compare the people who did and did not respond, and then describe in the paper what the differences were statistically. Many authors do not include that information. If they have not included it, then make a note of this potential weakness of the study.

Now take this same critical approach to reading about how the data were collected. Was a questionnaire or survey used? If so, what questions or items were included? Was research completed on the instrument itself before it was used in this study? For example, what do the authors report about the validity and reliability of the instrument? If data from a national study were used, then have the authors provided references so you can go back and get the information about how the data were collected? Do not automatically assume that a study was done correctly just because a national sample of subjects was drawn or this was part of a very large project. Read critically. Continue to read each part of the methods section of the paper in this way.

Results Section

Reread the purpose of the paper, and then examine the results section to see whether the authors answered the research questions or hypotheses they initially stated. Were additional questions posed and answered in the process of addressing the main questions? Were there additional research questions that were not answered?

Discussion Section

As you read the paper, think about the strengths and weaknesses of the study, and then note whether the authors described the same problems or advantages. Note especially what additional research questions were not addressed. Ask yourself what the implications of the results were or the significance of these findings.

References

You might find it useful to make notes about the references at the end of each paper. Specifically, go through the references of each paper and add to your own list (in the Source Documents Subfolder in Chapter 5) those that need follow-up.

(Continues)

EXHIBIT 5-1 How to Abstract a Research Paper (*Continued*)

Acknowledgments

This column topic might be included in the review if issues such as funding source are relevant. For example, you might consider whether the funding source of a research project posed a potential conflict of interest, such as a study about the rates of teenage smoking that has been funded by the tobacco industry.

Reviewer-Specific Topics

A Review Matrix should be tailored to the purpose of your review of the literature. Rarely will a review be so comprehensive as to include all of the column topics described here. In fact, you may choose to include only a few of the topics described previously and instead opt for some very specific topics of your own. For example, if your review of the literature is limited to experimental studies, then it might be redundant to have a column topic on experimental designs. Alternatively, if you believe that knowing which kinds of experimental designs would be important to understanding this literature, then you will need such a column topic. These reviewer-specific column topics may dominate the review of the literature, to the exclusion of many of the other topics listed.

Some General Advice

Rarely will you ever read straight through a paper in a linear fashion, from introduction to the discussion section. You may begin this way, but as you get into the paper, you will find it necessary to go back and recheck some of the details. For example, in the midst of the methods section you may jump ahead to the results section ("Did they really keep all of the subjects in the study who were enrolled at the beginning?") or in the middle of reading about the results, you may return to the introduction section ("What did the authors say the purpose was?"). As you read these papers, maintain a running dialogue with yourself about what the researchers intended to do, what they really did, what they reported they found, and what they actually found. This double-checking is important. Do not assume anything, and do not give any author of a research paper the benefit of the doubt. In reviewing the literature, the best attitude is to be methodologically suspicious and ever questioning.

Additional Information

In the meantime, as you read each source document, add to your list of references and download additional articles that will be added to the Source Documents Subfolder, as needed. Not everything will fit neatly under one of the column topics. If you are using a spreadsheet or the table option in a word processor to create the Review Matrix, insert new columns to include these notes. Expect to expand the number of columns in your Review Matrix.

FRINGE BENEFITS OF THE ABSTRACTING PROCESS

The reason for constructing a Review Matrix is to provide a structured basis for analyzing the literature and writing a review in the form of a narrative synthesis. Constructing a Review Matrix is both tedious and time consuming, but there are other advantages in the abstracting process itself, provided that you have done a thorough job of collecting the most relevant research papers on a subject. In the first place, you learn something about the sociology of the subject you are reviewing. Second, by taking apart and abstracting each study one at a time using the same set of column topics, you are better able to state questions of your own. Finally, you begin to have a better sense of what is missing and where new research is needed.

Sociology of the Research Topic

As you carefully read and abstract each source document in chronological order, especially if they are research papers in a specific area, you will begin to know the following:

- Who the researchers are and with whom they collaborate
- Where the research is being done (e.g., which country and which specific university)
- Whether they tend to use the same data sets
- What the funding sources are
- Which studies are cited repeatedly

In other words, without consciously trying to, you begin to become aware of the sociology of this research topic as you abstract the studies.

Who the Researchers Are

Knowing the names of the researchers is useful if you want to find related studies by running an author search on PubMed or one of the other electronic bibliographic databases. Science Citation Index is a useful source for finding additional studies by authors not included in the group that is now familiar to you. Knowing who collaborates with whom is important when learning about a new research field. For example, what appears to be simultaneous research efforts being done by a multitude of different researchers may, on closer inspection, be the product of the same group or subgroup of collaborators who happen to be located in diverse university and nonacademic settings. (For example, perhaps by one or two professors at one university in collaboration with their former students now at other universities or research labs or clinical settings.) There is nothing wrong with such an effort; in fact, it has become even more feasible with use of the Internet. Such information would be useful if you wanted to contact someone in that group and discovered that one of them was in your institution or a place nearby.

Where the Research Is Done

In the process of abstracting, you will begin to notice where the authors are located geographically. Some research efforts take place in a single university or institution; others, as suggested, may be spread throughout the country. For example, most of the initial research in evidence-based medicine was done at McMaster University in Ontario, Canada, although there were some collaborators in other Canadian and American universities. If you were interested in pursuing that topic in greater depth, going to McMaster or contacting someone there might be the first place to start. Checking out the group's website for a list of current or prospective publications would also be useful.

Data Sets They Have in Common

Often researchers in a related area use the same data set, such as one of the National Health Interview Surveys[2-4] or the National Health and Nutrition Examination Survey (NHANES). If you are familiar with how the data were gathered and what the strengths and limitations of these data sets are, then you are in a better position to evaluate the studies that used them. To locate studies based on these large-scale, nationally representative databases, use the database name, such as NHANES, as a key word search on PubMed or go to this website: http://www.cdc.gov/nchs/nhanes.htm.

Knowing which dataset was used might also help you decide to use one of those for your own research. Alternatively, you may choose some other dataset that might be more appropriate to your own research topic.

Funding Sources

If two or more studies have been funded by the same source, you might find research projects in the same area by looking up that funding source. For example, if a study has been funded by a research grant from the National Institute on Aging, search the National Institutes of Health database at http://www.nih.gov to see whether other studies or clinical trials have been funded. Some of the more recently funded studies may still be in progress, and the results will not yet have been published. It is also possible that some currently funded projects are being done by researchers other than those whose papers you have read, and they may be exploring different aspects of what is currently being published. In this case consider contacting the principal investigators of these ongoing studies to find out something about their work. Whether you choose to take this extra step depends on why you are doing this review of the literature. Many private foundations also list research projects they have funded in the past or are currently funding. Look them up on the Internet.

References Cited Repeatedly

When you are checking the references section at the end of most research papers published in health sciences journals, you may find that some of the research papers are being cited repeatedly by the authors of the documents you are abstracting. If you have not included these papers in your own review, consider adding them to the list you are abstracting.

Seeing What Is Missing

As you abstract each of the studies in your literature review, you are better able to develop your own questions about the research issues. Finding the answers to these questions will enable you to see the bigger picture. There is a real advantage for the person writing a synthesis or grant proposal to see where the holes are in the research on a topic. The abstracting process in the Review Matrix makes it possible for you to begin to see not only the issues that apparently have not been addressed but many of the methodological flaws as well. Discovering what is missing is part of owning the literature, and constructing the Review Matrix makes this possible.

Caroline's Quest: Constructing and Using a Review Matrix

After Caroline had arranged the reprints chronologically in the Source Documents Subfolder in her Documents Folder, she was ready to choose the column topics for the Review Matrix. She selected a random sample of these research papers, read them quickly, and jotted down further notes about which issues or topics appeared to be most important. She also reviewed the list of methodological topics that Professor Dickerson had given her. She knew that she would not need all of the methodological topics, but some of them probably would be useful.

Caroline began by listing the first three topics that were standard in every Review Matrix constructed using the Matrix Method: (1) authors, title, and journal; (2) year of publication; and (3) purpose. Next, she decided to concentrate on some of the methodological characteristics in her column topics, and for that reason she chose outcome variables, which she recorded as "dependent variables" in the Review Matrix. She knew that the studies varied in their definition of smoking. Depending on the purpose of each study, some authors concentrated only on cigarette smoking; others included chewing tobacco.

The next column topic she wrote was "independent variables." This was the topic that would help her sort out which characteristics the authors had used to look at variations in smoking behaviors. Caroline continued to add topics, such as the number of subjects in the study and whether the study was limited to females only or included both genders.

Caroline chose 17 topics, which she listed across the top of her still-blank Review Matrix. Eleven of those topics are shown in **Exhibit 5-2**, which lists only the methodological topics plus a comment topic that she reserved for making notes about the strengths and weaknesses of each study.

Caroline left several columns blank so she could add a few additional topics as she abstracted the studies. (If she was using the table option in Microsoft Word or an Excel file, then she would not have to leave any blank columns. Just choose Insert to insert a new column.) She was ready to begin abstracting the studies she had chosen.

Caroline began the abstracting process by setting aside the Review Matrix, taking out her calculator, selecting the yellow highlighter in her software, and turning to the first paper in the Source Documents Subfolder. This was the third time she had read this paper, but this was the most concentrated reading. Caroline highlighted a sentence in the purpose section of the paper and made a note of the

EXHIBIT 5-2 Caroline's Review Matrix for Research Literature on Smoking by Adolescent Girls

Authors, Title, Journal	Variables				Subjects				Data		Comments
	Year Pub	Purpose	Dependent Variable	Independent Variable	# of Subjects	Subject Characteristics	Sample Design	Source or Instrument	Year Data Collected		
Wang, Fitzhugh, Westerfield, Eddy. Family & peer influences on smoking behavior among American adolescents: an age trend. *J Adoles Health.*	1995	What is influence of family and peers on adolescent smoking?	Cigarette smoking only	Peer by sex family–sibling, father, mother	6,900	Male & female 14–18 yrs	Nat'l—random (82% response rate)	Nat'l Hlth Interv Surv	1988–89		• No response/ nonresp analysis for subjects • No info on data collect instrument • No race information

(*Continues*)

EXHIBIT 5-2 Caroline's Review Matrix for Research Literature on Smoking by Adolescent Girls (*Continued*)

	Variables				Subjects				Data	
Authors, Title, Journal	Year Pub	Purpose	Dependent Variable	Independent Variable	# of Subjects	Subject Characteristics	Sample Design	Source or Instrument	Year Data Collected	Comments
Altman, Levine, Coeytaux, Slade, Jaffe. Tobacco promotion and susceptibility to tobacco use among adol. Aged 12–17 years in a nationally repres. sample. *AJPH*.	1996	What is relation between youth susceptibility to tobacco use and participation in promotional campaign?	Use of tobacco. • Non-tobacco user • Sucep to tocacco • Current tobacco use • Use cigarette & chew tobacco	Age, gender, tobacco user in household, awareness of tobacco promot, know friend owns promot item, particip in tobacco promot, mail from tobacco free sample	1,047	Male & female, 12–17 yrs	Nat'l random (62% response rate)	Author conduct sample random digit dialing across U.S.	1993	• No resp/ nonresp analysis • No info on data collection instrument • No race info
French & Perry. Smoking among adolescent girls; prevalence & etiology. *JAMWA*.	1996	To review lit on prevalence & etiology of smok by adolescent girls.	Cigarette smoking	Female, race	Varies by study	Female, 17–18 years	Across multiple studies	Varies	Varies	Not an empirical study. Summary of literature only. • Info on race included. Note prevalence rates.

dependent and independent variables. She used her calculator to track the percentage of subjects who dropped out of the study or who did not respond to the survey. She also noted whether the authors provided a flowchart of number of subjects from recruitment to completion of study, as described in the CONSORT Guideline for designing better studies—described in Chapter 1. (See the CONSORT flowchart at this website: http://www.consort-statement.org/consort-statement /flow-diagram.) She did not have to repeat this flowchart, but could have a column labeled, Flowchart of Study Participants Included (yes/no). Caroline continued to read and reread the paper thoroughly until she had a clear understanding of what the purpose of the study was, how the authors had conducted the study, and what they had found.

Then Caroline turned to the Review Matrix and began to fill in the cells for that study under each of the column topics. After examining the list of references at the end of the paper, she added a few references to her list to look up in PubMed when she finished abstracting.

Caroline abstracted each paper immediately after reading it. Examples of three of the papers she abstracted, the Wang et al. study,[5] the Altman et al. paper,[6] and the French and Perry article,[7] are shown in Exhibit 5-2. Although the paper by French and Perry was not an actual study, it was important because it was a thorough review of the literature on the prevalence and etiology of smoking by adolescent girls and included 35 references that might provide further resources. Caroline included this paper and made a note in the comments column of her Review Matrix that the authors had reported rates of smoking for teenage girls.

After Caroline finished abstracting all the articles in Review Matrix, she saved it to the Review Matrix-CURRENT Subfolder. Next, she took the list of additional references she had compiled during the abstracting process and looked each up on PubMed. She then repeated the same process of considering whether to include any of these papers in her review and added a paper published in 1993. Caroline included this study in the Review Matrix at the end of the 1993 list and abstracted it as she had done the others. (She also added the PDF of the paper to the Source Documents Subfolder in the Documents Folder; see Chapter 4.)

After she was done, Caroline had a Review Matrix filled in with notes for each article. The matrix was a little messy because there were additional notes on yellow stickies and she had added a few more column topics. She was ready to write the synthesis.

What You Should Know or Be Able to Do by the End of This Chapter

The best test is whether you were able to follow the instructions for creating and using a Review Matrix is the Review Matrix itself.

1. Have you constructed a Review Matrix with columns to be used to abstract each source document?

2. Have you generated the names of the column topics by reading a sample of the articles and making decisions?

3. Have you arranged the source documents in your Review Matrix chronologically, from oldest at the beginning and most current at the end?

4. Have you completed the Review Matrix by abstracting the source documents, using the Rule of Rows?

5. If you added a new reference to abstract in your Review Matrix, did you also put a PDF of the new article in the Source Documents Subfolder in the Documents Folder, as well as in a separate row in the Review Matrix?

If you have done these five things, then you know or should be able to do what was taught in this chapter.

REFERENCES

1. Moher D, Liberati A, Tetzlaff J, Altman DG; The PRISMA Group. Preferred reporting items for systematic reviews and meta-analyses: the PRISMA Statement. *BMJ*. 2009;339:b2535. doi:http://dx.doi.org/10.1136/bmj.b2535.

2. National Center for Health Statistics. *Health Interview Survey Procedures, 1957–1974*. Hyattsville, MD: U.S. Department of Health, Education, and Welfare, Public Health Service, Health Resources Administration; 1975.

3. Kovar MG, Poe GS. *The National Health Interview Survey Design, 1975–83*. Hyattsville, MD: U.S. Department of Health and Human Services, Public Health Service, National Center for Health Statistics; 1985.

4. Masey JT, Moore TF, Parsons VL, Tadros W. *Design and Estimation for the National Health Interview Survey, 1985–94*. Hyattsville, MD: U.S. Department of Health and Human Services, Public Health Service, Centers for Disease Control, National Center for Health Statistics; 1989.

5. Wang MQ, Fitzhugh EC, Westerfield RC, Eddy JM. Family and peer influences on smoking behavior among American adolescents: an age trend. *J Adoles Health*. 1995;16:200-203.

6. Altman DG, Levine DW, Coeytaux R, Slade J, Jaffe R. Tobacco promotion and susceptibility to tobacco use among adolescents aged 12 through 17 years in a nationally representative sample. *Am J Public Health*. 1996;86:1590-1593.

7. French SA, Perry CL. Smoking among adolescent girls: prevalence and etiology. *J Am Med Womens Assoc*. 1996;51:25-28.

CHAPTER 6

Synthesis Folder: How to Use a Review Matrix to Write a Synthesis

The goal of a review of the literature is to summarize your critical analysis about the research literature on a specific topic in the form of a narrative synthesis. A narrative form means you will describe the results in words, not in a statistical form (such as a meta-analysis). The purpose of this chapter is to tell you and show you how to write a narrative synthesis based on the Review Matrix and the PRISMA Flowchart of Documents.[1] This chapter includes the following sections:

- What Is a Synthesis?
- How to Organize a Synthesis Folder
- How to Use a Review Matrix to Write a Synthesis
- How to Write a Synthesis of the Literature
- Finalizing the PRISMA Flowchart of Documents
- Examples: Use of the Matrix Method and PRISMA Flowchart in the Peer-Reviewed Literature
- Caroline's Quest: Writing a Synthesis
- What You Should Know or Be Able to Do by the End of This Chapter

WHAT IS A SYNTHESIS?

A synthesis is a critical analysis and review of the scientific literature on a specific topic and usually can take one of two major forms: a narrative synthesis or a meta-analysis synthesis. The purpose of this chapter is to describe how to write a

161

narrative synthesis based on critical analysis and integration of the studies in your final copy of the Review Matrix. A synthesis based on a meta-analysis is beyond the scope of this book. The narrative form of a synthesis written in words, represents a logical integration of the studies in your Review Matrix.

In the Matrix Method, a synthesis is based on peer-reviewed papers or source documents in your Review Matrix. You may have decided to include other kinds of documents; examples are editorials, summaries by distinguished groups of scientists such as the IOM, conference abstracts, or other forms of the grey literature. A synthesis describes the themes of the research as they have developed across the studies in your review and over the years, including similarities and differences in purpose, content, methodology, and findings. A synthesis also examines the source documents for what is missing—where the holes are in both the content and the research methodology. The goal of a synthesis is to analyze critically the content of the research, methodologies, and results and then to pull the disparate parts together into a logical, coherent narrative.

What Is NOT a Synthesis?

A simple summary of each of the research papers, whether the studies are in chronological form or in a matrix, is not a synthesis, nor is it even a review of the literature. A synthesis has to demonstrate your critical analysis of these papers and your ability to integrate the results.

Advantages of a Synthesis

Most people find that they do not formulate interpretations or opinions about the research studies until they have written a structured review of the literature. A well-written literature review requires that you complete two major tasks: critically analyze the literature and write a synthesis. The operational word here is *write*. To stop before putting the synthesis into written form will have accomplished only half the task of a literature review.

What This Chapter Does Not Cover

This chapter is not about how to write in general. There are excellent books available on that subject, beginning with the classic *If You Want to Write* by Brenda Ueland.[2] Other excellent guides are *How to Write: Advice and Reflections* by the Pulitzer Prize–winning writer Richard Rhodes,[3] and *Writing Down the Bones* by award-winning writing instructor Natalie Goldberg.[4] You must have a good grammar book. A classic is *The Elements of Style* by Strunk and White[5]; its witty, contemporary counterpart is *Woe Is I* by Patricia O'Conner.[6] These writing and grammar books are excellent resources, whether you intend to write a synthesis of the literature or any other kind of document.

HOW TO ORGANIZE A SYNTHESIS FOLDER

Your Synthesis Folder will have three subfolders. Set them up before you begin to write the synthesis of your literature review. These three subfolders are Synthesis-CURRENT Subfolder, Synthesis-PREVIOUS Subfolder, and Synthesis-FINAL Subfolder.

1. **Synthesis-CURRENT Subfolder**

   You need a subfolder that you can always go to at the beginning of each working session that contains your most recent draft of the synthesis. This subfolder satisfies that need. Label your first draft using the following: [current date] Synthesis. For example:

   06-10-2016 Synthesis.

   This file goes into the Synthesis-CURRENT Subfolder. Save your file often and again at the end of the working session.

   The next time you sit down to write, select the current document in the Synthesis-CURRENT Subfolder, make another copy using the "save as" option, and change the date of that file to the current date. For example:

   06-11-2016 Synthesis.

   The file with the most current date remains in the Synthesis-CURRENT Subfolder, and the older file (e.g., **06-10-2016** Synthesis, is now moved to the second folder, the Synthesis-PREVIOUS Subfolder).

   Now begin writing on the current version of the synthesis: **06-11-2016** Synthesis. There should be only one draft of your synthesis in your Synthesis-CURRENT Subfolder at any one time. Keep it tidy!

2. **Synthesis-PREVIOUS Subfolder**

   Save every copy of your synthesis by date until you have completed this final stage of writing a review of the literature. You may find it necessary to return to one of your earlier versions because your current copy may have become corrupted or you may have inadvertently erased an important part. For example, your most recent copy located in the Synthesis-PREVIOUS Subfolder is:

   06-10-2016 Synthesis

   and this may become very useful.

3. **Synthesis-FINAL Subfolder**

You need a place to put the final version of your synthesis; this is that subfolder. To do this, make a copy of the your most recent draft of the synthesis located in the Synthesis-CURRENT Subfolder, which by now is:

08-07-2016 Synthesis.

You may have completed your synthesis of the literature weeks or months ago, but by having this final version of the synthesis in this Synthesis-FINAL Subfolder, you will always know where to find it.

Incidentally, if this process of using CURRENT-PREVIOUS-FINAL Subfolders seems familiar, it is. You used the same process to save your copies of the Review Matrix documents, as described in Chapter 5. The Review Matrix and the synthesis are *the* most important files you generate in using the Matrix Method. Don't lose them.

HOW TO USE A REVIEW MATRIX TO WRITE A SYNTHESIS

The Tools You Will Need: Review Matrix, Source Documents, and PRISMA Flowchart

After you have abstracted all the source documents in your Review Matrix and stored a current copy in your Review Matrix-CURRENT Subfolder (see Chapter 5), you are ready to begin to draft the synthesis. You will use not only the content in the matrix, but also the original peer-reviewed papers in the Source Documents Subfolder (see Chapter 4). Thus, you will need both the most current copy of your Review Matrix and the source documents on your desktop when you write the synthesis. Later in this process, you will add the most current copy of the PRISMA Flowchart[1] (see Chapter 4) to the methods section in your synthesis.

The Rule of Columns

The Review Matrix has a different use for writing a synthesis than it did for abstracting source documents. Constructing the Review Matrix required you follow the "Rule of Rows" to develop each row of the matrix by analyzing one study at a time based on the column topics.

When writing a synthesis of the literature, however, you will integrate the information down the columns of the Review Matrix as you compare the studies.

This is what I call the "Rule of Columns." Thus, in creating a Review Matrix, you use the Rule of Rows to abstract each paper, but in writing a synthesis, you use the Rule of Columns. It is important to remember these two rules when using the Matrix Method.

Of course you have to know the studies as you begin to write the synthesis, but you are now looking at these source documents from a different perspective. For example, you could think about how the studies varied over time in their use of a particular theory. Alternatively, you might want to identify only those studies that included both male and female subjects. By scanning a particular column of the Review Matrix, you can readily identify those studies. (It might be easier to sort the studies in your Review Matrix on the basis of information in one of the columns. This sorting task is especially easy if you set up your Review Matrix using either the table option in a Word document or as an Excel file.)

You might also look for the lack of something across the studies. For example, in papers on the epidemiology of epilepsy, did any of the subject populations include individuals who were 65 years of age or older? If you abstracted information in the Review Matrix about the subjects' age ranges, you will be able to look for that possibility. In general, as you critically evaluate the different studies, think about underlying factors that show variations, or lack thereof, over time or before/after a groundbreaking paper.

Why Are You Doing This Review?

The first step in actually writing a synthesis is to be clear with yourself about *why* you are doing a literature review. The most common reasons include summarizing previous scholarly work for a paper or report for a class; gathering background material for a presentation or publication; preparing a thesis or dissertation required in a graduate program; writing a research proposal requesting grant or contract funds; or developing a manuscript of a scientific paper, possibly based on your own research or that of others.

Where you describe the literature review in your final paper and its *focus* will depend on why you are doing it. In a thesis or dissertation, the previous research section contains most of the review of the literature; whereas, in a standard grant or contract proposal, the background and significance sections usually include most of the literature review.

In a thesis or dissertation and a research proposal, the review of the literature may focus not only on the major topic, for example, previous research on the effects of poor nutrition among low-income children, but also on a methodological review, such as, the types of research methods used by previous researchers in the field to investigate that topic over time.

In a scientific paper in a peer-reviewed journal publication in the health sciences, the review of the literature will be most evident in the introduction section. Thus, the purpose of the review may dictate its focus and where you put it in your final paper.

HOW TO WRITE A SYNTHESIS OF THE LITERATURE

Define the Purpose of the Review

The first step in actually writing a synthesis is to define clearly the purpose of the review of the literature. You should have done this already when you began assembling the Paper Trail Folder; however, that purpose may have changed as you read and reread the source documents. Perhaps the purpose is more refined in scope or has been expanded to encompass more issues. Either way, the first working sentence of your synthesis should be this: "The purpose of this review of the literature is . . . ."

Describe the Search Strategy

Describe briefly the final search strategy you used to select and review the documents included in your literature review. Be sure to include the date of the final search strategy. This description provides basic information about your search and selection process, such as the period of time covered by the review, sources used (including electronic bibliographic databases and journals), types of articles (such as empirical papers or abstracts from scientific conferences, etc.), and inclusions and exclusions for selecting source documents at different stages of the review. The following fictional example based on your numbers of documents in the PRISMA Flowchart[1] conveys this information:

The review of the literature covered a 10-year period, from 2006 to 2016. As documented in the PRISMA Flowchart,[1] the final date of the search strategy was January 5, 2016. The search included the use of three electronic bibliographic databases, MEDLINE, PsycInfo, and International Pharmaceutical Abstracts, with special attention to the leading clinical journals in this area (*Journal of X, Journal of Y,* and *Journal of Z*). Only empirical studies were reviewed; letters to the editor, policy statements, and program descriptions were excluded. A total of 115 papers was examined, of which 21 met the inclusion/exclusion criteria.

Because you are using the Matrix Method, you also will need to reference this book and describe what topics were used to abstract the documents. Here is an example of that narrative section of your review:

Using the Matrix Method,[7] each of the 21 papers was evaluated in ascending chronological order using a Review Matrix with 12 column topics: journal identification, purpose, definition of independent and dependent variables, covariates, methodological design, sampling design, number of subjects, respondent–nonrespondent analysis, data sources, validity and reliability of data collection, results, and significance.

The description of the search and abstracting process will vary, depending on your purpose. For example, if you are reviewing the literature for a research paper, the description may need to be more detailed. Regardless of the purpose of your review, a statement of the search and abstracting process will give the reader a sense of the thoroughness of your literature review.

List the Principal Sections of the Synthesis

Now think about which topics you will use to organize the synthesis. A thorough synthesis of the literature includes a discussion of *each* of the following:

- Issues and Research Question: Describe the major reasons or problems that motivated this body of research, including the theoretical or conceptual models and the hypothesis or research question.
- Methods: Summarize the research methods used to investigate the problems, including the column topics, the methodological designs, data collection instruments and procedures, subjects, and data analysis. (Go back

and review the section on the Methods Map in Chapter 2.) Most authors of empirical studies put the final PRISMA Flowchart[1] in the methods section of their narrative synthesis.

- Results: List the major findings of your literature review or results or the answers to each of the questions you stated for your paper. Consider restating each research question, followed by the results from the studies.

- Missing or inadequate topics: Describe the topics or issues that you have identified as missing, that is, those that have not been investigated at all or those that have been covered inadequately.

- Critical analysis: Describe your critical analysis of each of these sections.

It is important to separate your discussion of the literature (i.e., the issues, methods, results, and missing topics) from your critical analysis. Make certain that you specify which is which in your review. Although all five sections of your synthesis are needed, your critical analysis of this body of research is probably the most important. Critical, in this context, is not the same as negative. A critical analysis is one in which you have weighed all the evidence and made an informed judgment about the adequacy, appropriateness, and thoroughness of the studies reviewed.

You can structure the written synthesis of the literature in several different ways. One approach is to write up each of the first four sections—issues, methods, missing or inadequate, and results—and at the end of each section give a critical analysis.

Another approach is to summarize the first four topics together and conclude with a critical analysis. Often the decision about how to structure a review of the literature will be made after you have written the first draft, not at the beginning of the process. In fact, you might choose the structure only after you revise the synthesis several times.

Alternatively, the reason for doing the literature review may dictate the structure and format of your synthesis. For example, a synthesis written for a doctoral dissertation will be very different from one prepared for a research study manuscript being submitted to a peer-reviewed journal.

Critically Analyze, Then Synthesize Information in the Review Matrix

With the purpose and structure of your narrative synthesis in mind, how do you use the Review Matrix to synthesize the information? Read each of the matrix columns from top to bottom and determine what happened within each column topic across the studies and over time. For example, if you are summarizing the themes of the research studies, look down the purpose column in the Review Matrix. Are there specific issues that appear, disappear, and then reappear over the years?

If it is necessary to gather more details, go back and reread some of the papers, which you already will have arranged in convenient, chronological order in the Source Documents Subfolder. Having abstracted all of the articles, you should have developed a sense of how thoroughly the various authors reviewed other studies by their inclusion of citations to published papers. Did these authors refer to other studies? Alternatively, did other authors seem to strike out on their own, without referring to the work of previous research that could have been used to better develop their own ideas? Taken as a body of research, does this collection of articles suggest that many different themes were addressed over the period you reviewed, or does this set of articles focus on one central theme, with the studies building on one another?

Do the papers seem to concentrate on increasingly specific details about the same issue, with only a few that explore new areas of inquiry? Is this an appropriate, creative, or necessary diversion from the mainstream research on the subject? If you are developing ideas for your own research, perhaps in the form of a dissertation or research proposal, what holes are there that you might focus on in this body of research? If you find a something that is missing in your review of the literature, use that topic as a key word in PubMed to double-check that you might have overlooked the very study that focused on that "hole." If you are going to claim that something is missing, then you had better be extra careful that it is indeed missing in the literature and not just missing in your review of the literature!

The same kind of thinking could be applied to the methodological designs used to examine the research questions. You might want to sort the Review Matrix on the basis of experimental, quasi-experimental, pre-experimental, and observational designs, and then write your narrative for studies using each of those designs. But this can be a problem if the authors used two or more research questions, each with a different methodological design. Do what is most logical for your review of the literature.

You also might ask yourself whether the studies were merely descriptive, or did subsequent studies describe innovative approaches for solving the problem? For example, in the research literature on falls among older women, initial papers described high prevalence rates that often resulted in the women's confinement to a nursing home or in their death. Later papers reported a statistical association between falls and use of antianxiety drugs, with the conclusion that these medications were overused in the older population. In subsequent papers, only a subclass of antianxiety drugs was found to be associated with loss of balance, which increased the likelihood of falls. Next was a series of studies that described the effects of different methods for intervening with practicing physicians to convince them to change their prescription of these drugs, especially for older people. Taken as a whole, this body of research moved from the initial description of the problem, through association with risk factors, to intervention. The corresponding methodological designs used in these studies followed a similar progression from descriptive to quasi-experimental to experimental designs.

FINALIZING THE PRISMA FLOWCHART OF DOCUMENTS

As part of the methods section in writing the synthesis, describe the number of documents you identified from the initial search to the final selection. You may have started with over a thousand documents in your initial stage, but by the time you get to the point of critically analyzing source documents for your Review Matrix, you have only 25 source documents. You will be using an adaption of the PRISMA Flowchart for Documents Through Different Phases of the Review[1] to track these numbers. Be sure to provide a citation for the source of the PRISMA Flowchart[1] in your synthesis.

Tracking the number of documents is an important part of a literature review. Together with your statement about the search parameters that generated your numbers, reporting your adaptation of the PRISMA Flowchart[1] gives the reader a sense of your commitment to verification and reproducibility of what you have done. In making this statement, be sure to describe the date of the final run. That is your way of saying that after that final date, you can no longer be held responsible for any papers published afterwards.

EXAMPLES: USE OF THE MATRIX METHOD AND PRISMA FLOWCHART IN THE PEER-REVIEWED LITERATURE

Sometimes it helps to see an example of a review of the literature using the Matrix Method, and how the PRISMA Flowchart[1] is incorporated in that review. In this section, I describe three papers published recently in the peer-reviewed nursing literature. Your task is to go into PubMed, obtain a PDF of each of these papers, and follow along with me as I focus only on their use of the Matrix Method[7] and the PRISMA Flowchart.[1] These are the papers I will discuss:

1. Guo Q, Jacelon CS. An integrative review of dignity in end-of-life care. *Palliative Med.* 2014;28(7):931-940.[8]
2. Nielsen AH, Angel S. How diaries written for critically ill influence the relatives: a systematic review of the literature. *Nurs Crit Care.* 2016;21(2):88-96. doi:10.1111/nicc.12158.[9]
3. Choi M, De Gagne JC. Autonomy of nurse practitioners in primary care: An integrative review. *J Am Assoc Nurse Pract.* 2016;28:170-174. doi:10.1002/2327-6924.12288.[10]

Although the papers are similar in their use of the Matrix Method to analyze the source documents, only one[9] included the Review Matrix in the paper, another[10] made the Review Matrix available at the publisher's website, and the third[8] described the column topics of the Review Matrix and subdivision of the source documents based on the authors' predetermined conceptual classification, but did not make the Review Matrix available. All three ways of handling the Review Matrix in a published paper are appropriate.

In a Master's thesis or doctoral dissertation, you might want to include the Review Matrix in your Methods section, together with the PRISMA Flowchart of source documents at different stages of the literature review.

The other characteristics the three papers had in common were the following:

- The purpose or aim of the study was clearly defined in *both* the Abstract and the Introduction sections of the paper.
- A description of each paper was clearly stated in the Introduction section as either an integrative[8,10] or a systematic[9] review of the literature.
- A concise review of the literature was included in the Introduction or Background section to support the purpose of the paper.
- The electronic data bases used, e.g., PubMed, CINAHL, PsycINFO, to gather source documents were stated specifically.
- The use of quantitative and qualitative source documents was clearly described in all three papers.

- The PRISMA Flowchart[1] and the Matrix Method[7] were in either the methods or analytic strategy sections; all papers included the numbers of source documents in the flowchart at different stages of the review.

The papers differed in the content of the review, the peer-reviewed journals in which they were published, and the universities in which the authors were based.

There are other papers describing the use of the Matrix Method in the peer reviewed literature in the health sciences, but these three provide excellent examples of how a narrative synthesis based on the combined use of the Matrix Method[7] and the PRISMA Flowchart[1] are presented in the context of an empirical paper that includes qualitative and quantitative source documents and a synthesis of the literature.

Caroline's Quest: Writing a Synthesis

Caroline met with Professor Dickerson to go over her Review Matrix and discuss the next steps.

"Keep in mind why you are writing this synthesis," Professor Dickerson cautioned her. "The way you write the review, its length, and the issues you cover may vary depending on whether the synthesis is being written for a term paper, a thesis, or a grant proposal. In this case, you know it is the introductory section for your thesis, but in the future your purpose may vary."

Caroline understood his point but had a question about her immediate task. "I'd like to talk about how to organize the synthesis itself. You know, what do I discuss first, then next, and so forth?"

Professor Dickerson nodded and said, "I know what you mean. The first thing to remember is that you should not merely summarize each paper one at a time. That is not a review of the literature. Instead, think about the issues you want to describe. Certainly you will be providing information about each study, but your focus should be on a critical analysis of the major aspects of research that these studies cover. You might begin your synthesis by describing the purpose of your review and limitations that you chose, such as a focus on adolescent girls between the ages of 13 and 18 years. You could also include a few sentences on the search strategy itself, the years you restricted it to, the databases you searched, and the number of articles you included at each stage of the review. Use your PRISMA Flowchart[1] to chart these numbers of documents. All of this is preliminary to your actual writing of the synthesis, however, and should probably not take more than a page. Concentrate the remainder of your synthesis on the critical analysis of the studies.

"For example," he continued, "think about the different kinds of research questions that the authors asked in their studies. Were there any major themes? If so, describe them briefly. Summarize the major findings, and then discuss how the studies differed in what they found. In general, think about using the following strategy: summarize the issue, describe variations across the studies, discuss the strengths and weaknesses of the studies, and give your interpretation about what this means."

Caroline looked at the materials she had brought with her. "So how do I use the Review Matrix in writing the synthesis?" she asked. "Or is preparing the Review Matrix just a way of making me read each article in a disciplined fashion?"

"Good question," Professor Dickerson laughed. "You're right. Filling in the Review Matrix does make you read each study carefully and make notes on the same set of topics, but the Review Matrix is also very useful in two other ways in the actual writing of the synthesis. The matrix helps you think about which topics to cover in the synthesis. The organization of the synthesis you write will not be identical to the column topics listed across the top of your Review Matrix, but those column topics may help you in thinking about which issues to include."

Professor Dickerson pointed to Caroline's Review Matrix on her laptop. "But the second and most practical way to use the Review Matrix is to read down each column and think about how the studies vary or how they are alike. For example, look at the variations in number of subjects across the studies."

Caroline reexamined the Review Matrix she had prepared and began to see the variations Professor Dickerson was talking about. "I hadn't realized how much the studies differed," she commented. "At first they all looked pretty much alike. Actually, when I began doing this review of the literature, I had the sense that there was nothing left to study. It seemed like all of the research questions had been asked and answered."

Professor Dickerson smiled and replied, "Yes, that's the sense most people have when they first begin to read the scientific literature on a specific topic. By constructing a Review Matrix, however, you begin to see where the holes are. The Review Matrix helps you realize which areas appear to be missing and which topics have been covered pretty thoroughly.

"But it is important," he cautioned, "if you see what you think is an area or aspect that is missing, then try to find other studies in which the missing topic has been studied. In other words, is it missing because no one has studied that aspect of the field, or is it because you didn't do a thorough enough job of finding all the studies? You will find yourself adding a few more source documents at this stage of the review process. If you do add a document, then use the Rule of Rows to fill out the cells for that study."

"Okay, I understand," Caroline looked at her professor and continued in a firm voice, "But this afternoon, I have to write the first draft of the synthesis for my thesis. What do I begin with? Then what do I write next? How do I organize this synthesis?"

Professor Dickerson took out a blank sheet of paper and made some notes as he talked. "Keep in mind that the organization will vary depending on your purpose. But as we discussed before, one structure you might use is the following: describe the purpose of your literature review; briefly summarize the characteristics of the search process and include your adaptation of the PRISMA Flowchart[1] here. In the next section, reference the Matrix Method[7] and describe the structure you are going to follow in writing this synthesis—in other words, the topics you are going to summarize; discuss the similarities and differences across the studies under each topic; and finally, describe your interpretation of what this means. In your interpretation, state your opinion, based on your logical and critical analysis of the literature in the Review Matrix. Include a copy of your Review Matrix at this point. Summarize your thoughts about what is known based on this research, what hasn't been adequately covered, and what is missing. If you have some suggestions about how you would address these inadequacies, then describe them. In writing the section on your interpretation, be sure to make it clear that these are your opinions and not those of the authors of the papers."

Caroline gathered together her papers and prepared to leave. "I feel that I really know this literature now," she said. "Well, I have a good sense of what this set of articles covers, anyway," she amended. "For me, the Review Matrix was most helpful in making me concentrate on the same set of topics in reading each paper."

Professor Dickerson nodded and replied, "You'll also find that the Review Matrix is very helpful in the writing process too if you use the Rule of Columns. I'll be interested in seeing how your first draft of the synthesis turns out."

What You Should Know or Be Able to Do by the End of This Chapter

By the end of Chapter 6, you should be able to explain these concepts to a person who is reading this book for the first time:

1. What is a synthesis of the literature?
2. What is *not* a synthesis of the literature?
3. How do you use the Review Matrix to critically evaluate the literature?
4. What are the Rules of Rows and Columns and how is each rule applied to the Review Matrix?
5. What are the different sections you will write in a synthesis of the literature?
6. Describe several ways you can adapt the PRISMA Flowchart to show how you might track the number of documents from the beginning to the end of your review.
7. Do you have to include your Review Matrix (complete with all rows and columns) if you submit your final review for publication in a peer-reviewed journal?
8. Now that you are a teacher of the Matrix Method with these first seven items, include a copy of your synthesis here to demonstrate what you actually did.

REFERENCES

1. Moher D, Liberati A, Tetzlaff J, Altman DG; The PRISMA Group. Preferred reporting items for systematic reviews and meta-analyses: the PRISMA Statement. *BMJ*. 2009;339:b2535. doi:http://dx.doi.org/10.1136/bmj.b2535.
2. Ueland B. *If You Want to Write: A Book about Art, Independence and Spirit*. Reprint of 1938 in 2012 as an eBook edition. New York: Start Publishing; 2012.
3. Rhodes R. *How to Write: Advice and Reflections*. New York: William Morrow and Company; 1996.
4. Goldberg N. *Writing Down the Bones: Freeing the Writer Within*. 30th ed. New York: Shambhala Library; 2016.
5. Strunk W, White EB. *The Elements of Style*. 4th ed. New York: Longman Publisher; 1999.
6. O'Conner PT. *Woe Is I: The Grammarphobe's Guide to Better English in Plain English*. 3rd ed. New York: Riverhead Books; 2009.
7. Garrard J. *Health Sciences Literature Review Made Easy: The Matrix Method*. 5th ed. Burlington, MA: Jones & Bartlett Learning Publishers; 2017.

8. Guo Q, Jacelon CS. An integrative review of dignity in end-of-life care. *Palliative Med.* 2014;28(7):931-940.

9. Nielsen AH, Angel S. How diaries written for critically ill influence the relatives: a systematic review of the literature? *Nurs Crit Care.* 2016;21(2):88-96. doi: 10.1111/nicc.12158.

10. Choi M, De Gagne JC. Autonomy of nurse practitioners in primary care: An integrative review. *J Am Assoc Nurse Pract.* 2016;28:170-174. doi:10.1002/2327-6924.12288.

Applications Using the Matrix Method

Part III is about different ways to use the Matrix Method after you have produced your first Review Matrix and written your first narrative synthesis.

In Part III you will learn how to use multiple Master Folders (Chapter 7), how to implement a more sophisticated Matrix Indexing System (Chapter 8), and how to apply the Matrix Method in different health sciences settings (Chapter 9), and (by way of Caroline's Quest) how to use the Matrix Method in a nonhealth sciences application.

Appendix A provides you with a handy list of useful resources for literature reviews. Appendix B will be especially useful as you set up your folders and sub-folders in the Matrix Method.

With Appendix C, my publisher and I provide you with a departure from any other chapters or appendices in this book. This is an opportunity for digital exploration. Appendix C is about data visualization—its history, current uses, and applications that you can use now and in the future. You can enter this digital environment online by using the Online Access Code that is unique to your copy of this book. Enjoy!

CHAPTER 7

A Library of Master Folders

Creating a Master Folder is a first step in the Matrix Method, but if you have conducted literature reviews for two or more different subjects, then how do you manage multiple Master Folders? The purpose of this chapter is to describe what a library of Master Folders is and why it is worth developing and maintaining. The concept, which is simple, gives you efficiency to buy yourself time in the future. The Matrix Method tells you how to conduct a review of the literature; this chapter tells you what to do after the synthesis has been written. The sections of this chapter are as follows:

- What Is a Library of Master Folders?
- How to Create a Library of Master Folders
- How to Use a Library of Master Folders
- Making the Most of the Matrix Method
- Caroline's Quest: Building Her Own Library of Master Folders

WHAT IS A LIBRARY OF MASTER FOLDERS?

Suppose that over the past few years you have completed not one, but five, literature reviews on different subjects. For each of these literature reviews, you have created a complete Master Folder with the four folders described earlier in this book (i.e., Paper Trail Folder, Documents Folder, Review Matrix Folder, and Synthesis Folder). You now have a library of Master Folders consisting of a collection of computer folders on your desktop. Even one Master Folder makes a library. Just storing Master Folders, however, is not sufficient. This resource is useful only if two additional conditions are met: (1) the Master Folders are updated periodically, and (2) you create and use some kind of indexing system so you know what is available. The purpose of this chapter is to describe how to use a collection of Master Folders. The next chapter will describe the indexing system you may want to use.

Advantages of a Library of Master Folders

If you organize your Master Folders as a library, you buy yourself time, which can be a scarce resource, whether you are a student, researcher, or professional writer. With a Master Folders library, you also gain the practical advantage of not having to duplicate previous efforts to find and download a copy of an article or source document. In the initial review of the literature, you make a one-time investment of time and effort. By creating and maintaining a library of Master Folders, you will benefit from the interest on that investment in the future.

HOW TO CREATE A LIBRARY OF MASTER FOLDERS

A literature review is usually done in a flurry of activity, with an intense effort focused on getting the synthesis written and the product produced, whether it is a paper, a grant proposal, or a final report. Afterward, the by-products of this effort are set aside—the notes in the Paper Trail Folder, the downloaded articles in the Documents Folder, the Review Matrix in its folder, and the final written product in the Synthesis Folder. They are accumulated in the Master Folder until they are needed again. Usually the impetus for returning to a Master Folder is the need for a particular source document that you know was part of the initial review.

Adopt a Labeling Convention

The secret to being efficient in the future is knowing where your Master Folders are and keeping them up to date. Your first task is to assign a label to each of your Master Folders. For example, create a label based on the subject of your literature review: Epilepsy Master Folder or HIV/AIDS Master Folder. Next, store them all together in a folder of Master Folders. You might call this folder your Master Folders Library.

Take this labeling of folders one step further by using the same label for the four folders that make up the Master Folder. For example, in the Epilepsy

Master Folder, create an Epilepsy Paper Trail Folder, an Epilepsy Documents Folder, an Epilepsy Review Matrix Folder, and an Epilepsy Synthesis Folder. By using the same label, you can search your documents just on the label alone to find them all.

Keep the Master Folders Up to Date

Keeping your Master Folders up to date is another practice that takes time and self-discipline. As you come across new studies, download a copy of the article to the Source Documents Subfolder in the Documents Folder in the appropriate Master Folder. An alternative is to let new documents accumulate in a safe place, and at some later time file them in the Source Documents Subfolder in the appropriate Master Folders.

Expanding a Documents Folder is not the only reason for updating a Master Folder. Additions to the Paper Trail Folder might include new topical websites or lecture notes from subsequent courses or conferences. Consider setting aside one part of the Paper Trail Folder to store notes from scientific meetings you attended after the synthesis was written. You do not have to know exactly how you will use these added materials in the future, but you need a dependable storage system so you can find them when you need them. A library of updated Master Folders provides such a system.

HOW TO USE A LIBRARY OF MASTER FOLDERS

An updated library of Master Folders can be very useful as you progress through your academic or professional career. Simply finding things is a fundamental problem; trying to find things you know you have but cannot lay your hands on is a frustrating problem. A library of Master Folders provides a permanent storage system that you can use from course to course and year to year.

A second use for your library of Master Folders is integrating information across topics or content areas. Whether you are a graduate student, researcher, policy analyst, or writer, you will inevitably find yourself doing more than one review of the literature. Even when your literature review is on a single topic, you may find it necessary to delve into several different subjects, possibly with a review and synthesis of each.

For example, if you are conducting research on the effects of penicillin as a treatment for ear infections in children, you might need to review the literature on the clinical effectiveness of penicillin, later conduct a separate review on the epidemiology of ear infections, and still later do a third review of papers on research methodologies used to study patient outcomes of clinical treatment of ear infections. For each of these topics you could create a separate Master Folder, especially if the review has a complex paper trail or a large number of source documents in the Documents Folder. Your review of studies on the treatment of ear infections then might result in three Master Folders—one labeled Peds Ear Infect (Penicillin); a second, Peds Ear Infect (Epi); and a third, Peds Ear Infect (Res Mtds).

After you complete a synthesis on penicillin treatment, you might use the Master Folder on research methods as your central file for methodological papers and notes. Thus, a Master Folder that you created for one review could be useful in a multitude of other reviews.

A library of Master Folders that has been kept up to date can be a valuable resource for a group of people, such as a research team or collaborators on a project. A library can serve as a central archive, making it easier for team members to store and find commonly used materials. This also has the advantage of increasing the opportunity for shared knowledge. Let the rules for keeping the library up to date be simple; anyone can add an article or source document to the appropriate Master Folder in the library, but the same person also has to assume the responsibility of notifying other team members about the new addition by posting it in an indexing system on a server or updating the Source Documents Subfolder in the Documents Folder. A central archive buys time and effort for the team and reduces the necessity of downloading multiple copies and storing them in each individual's Master Folder.

MAKING THE MOST OF THE MATRIX METHOD

By now you probably understand the basic concepts about how to use the Matrix Method. But bear in mind that a successfully completed review of the literature may not always exactly follow the instructions in this textbook. **Exhibit 7-1** describes some of the concepts and the variations that may be useful to experienced users of the Matrix Method. These are given in the form of Frequently Asked Questions (FAQs) about how to get the most out of the Matrix Method.

EXHIBIT 7-1 FAQs About Getting the Most Out of the Matrix Method

Why Do I Have to Read an Article Multiple Times in the Matrix Method?

You read for different purposes. You need to read an article or source document up to three times. Here is a summary of each reading (and the chapters that describe the purpose for each).

- **First Reading: Select Document**. The first time you read a source document (an article or paper in a journal) is to decide whether it is relevant to your topic. This initial reading may be just of the abstract or a skimming of the article. For example, read the title and abstract in the bibliographic database (e.g., PubMed) to determine relevancy to your topic. You may select or discard potential articles at this stage, but try to be as broad in your choices as possible. This first reading does not have to be in chronological order by publication date. The end product is a set of downloaded articles or PDF files in your Source Documents Subfolder. See Chapter 4 about how to select documents for your review.
- **Second Reading: Identify Column Topics**. This reading is for the purpose of deciding what column topics to include in the Review Matrix. By this point you have selected a sample of journal articles (or other source documents). Organize them in chronological order, from oldest to most recent, and begin this reading with the oldest document. Reread the abstract and the entire article, making a list of potential column topics as you go. The end product at this stage is an empty Review Matrix with column topics listed across the top (and room for more to be added). See Chapter 5 about how to choose column topics for a Review Matrix.
- **Third Reading: Conduct a Critical Review**. At this stage, you read each article thoroughly and abstract it based on the column topics. This reading includes all source documents selected for your review of the literature, whether you have read them once or twice before. This is your first critical review of the article, and you approach it with a calculator and electronic sticky notes or other ways of making notes in the document itself. Read the article section by section and make notes in the cells of the Review Matrix (as well as copious notes on the article itself as you record your thoughts). The end product should be a filled-in Review Matrix with the column topics across the top and all the articles listed in chronological order (oldest to most recent) down the side. See Chapter 5 about how to analyze documents in a Review Matrix.
- **Later Readings: Compare**. A fourth, fifth, and sixth reading may be necessary as you develop your understanding of the literature you are reviewing. These later readings may be necessary as you compare an article with others. These comparisons could be about the purpose of the study, the

(Continues)

EXHIBIT 7-1 FAQs About Getting the Most Out of the Matrix Method
(*Continued*)

---

number of subjects who completed the treatment, or the authors' interpretation of the significance of the findings. While drawing these comparisons, you are creating the first draft of your synthesis. See Chapter 6
about how to use a Review Matrix to write a synthesis.

How Many Articles Are Enough?

This is a common question, and my answer is always the same: "It depends." You need to abstract enough articles that you feel you own the
literature. If only a few papers have been published about your topic,
then this may be a signal that you need to broaden your topic. If there are
too many (e.g., 100 or more), then narrow your focus, perhaps by selecting only studies with more stringent methodological designs (such as only
those with an experimental design or those with more than 25 subjects
in a group). If you are examining studies of a specific drug treatment and
there are too few published, then consider whether this drug is one of a
broader class of drugs. Including more publications about the treatment
effects of that broader class may help put this drug into perspective.

**How Far Back Do I Go in the Literature and When Do I Use an Old
Article?**

While you are reviewing abstracts in the selection process (the first reading), pay close attention to which publications those articles are refer-
encing. As you become more familiar with research papers about your
topic, it is likely that you will notice that some of the same authors are
referenced repeatedly by others. Conduct an author search in your bibliographic database (e.g., PubMed), identify which of each of the author's papers are related to your topic, and look at the dates of those
publications. If the dates are older than the ones you have included thus
far, then include them, and let the oldest of these be designated as your
oldest publication.

Sometimes it is possible to recognize frequently referenced authors
before the abstracting process begins, and the search for papers about
those can be started before you develop your Review Matrix. That is the
preferred strategy and allows you to begin the abstracting process from
a logical beginning. If not, be alert for frequently referenced authors

and include them at whatever stage of the abstracting process you discover them.

A related problem is when you find a paper in the peer-reviewed literature that is quite old compared to the papers you have already selected. If that really old paper is closely related to your topic, then consider the possibility that there are other papers you haven't found yet in between the oldest date and the date your other papers begin. Go back and look for them; perhaps this is the point to try using the Science Citation Index based on a search under each author's name. If you don't find any papers in between the two dates, then perhaps there are none, but include that oldest paper anyway.

What Do I Do About Qualitative Studies?

A qualitative study can be thought of as one that does not include statistical analysis, mainly because the results do not lend themselves to quantitative procedures. Qualitative results can have a powerful impact on the interpretation of data that cannot be gathered any other way. For example, if a researcher is studying the impact of a new federal policy on quality of life of nursing home elderly, then one kind of study would be to ask nursing home residents about the positive and negative aspects of living there. Do this before and after the policy has been implemented. A comparison of responses from both periods may be very useful. Another example would be a content analysis of interview data in qualitative research about treatment effects of a new medical device. A content analysis can be a rigorous nonquantitative method for systematically examining variations in interview data. See an example of the use of content analysis in a study my colleagues and I did of organizational change in the management of hepatitis C.[1]

If some of the articles describe qualitative research and others quantitative research, should they be included in the same Review Matrix? How do we draw conclusions from such a mixture of quantitative and qualitative research? There is no definite rule about this. My tendency would be to separate the quantitative and qualitative studies, use the same column headings if possible, and then add new ones for the qualitative studies. Examples of column topics that would be the same for both might be number of subjects, data collection instrument, validity and

(*Continues*)

EXHIBIT 7-1 FAQs About Getting the Most Out of the Matrix Method
                  (*Continued*)

---

reliability studies of data collection instrument, sampling method, and methodological design. New columns to be added for the qualitative studies might include details about how data were collected (e.g., focus group, telephone interview) and how data were analyzed).

In writing the synthesis, examine the results of the two review matrices (quantitative and qualitative research) separately. You may find that one complements or enriches the other. Alternatively, combine all the studies in a single, chronologically arranged Review Matrix, regardless of quantitative or qualitative characteristics, and summarize these results.

In general, as research methods have become more sophisticated over time, many scientists use both kinds of research, and it is very difficult to characterize a study as solely quantitative or qualitative.

How Do I Review and Abstract Longitudinal Studies?

Longitudinal studies are those that collect data from subjects at multiple points over a long period of time, where researchers can define *long* in different ways, such as multiple weeks, months, or years.

Publications about longitudinal studies can vary in several ways; the primary author may differ, the research site may not be the same, the research question may vary around a principal topic, the purpose of the paper may change (e.g., some may describe new methodological developments, whereas others may concentrate on clinical outcomes), and the year of publication of the paper varies over time. If all of these studies clearly show that there was a core research team with a primary research goal, then try this suggestion for abstracting these studies. Set aside a section of the Review Matrix and abstract the longitudinal journal articles in their chronological order (from oldest to most recent) using the same column topics as in the rest of your Review Matrix. This arrangement will give you the opportunity to consider that subset of research as a whole rather than as a collection of discrete studies that happened to have some commonalities. If there are multiple longitudinal studies, perhaps from researchers based in different universities or different countries, then you will be in a better position to describe these research endeavors as a group and perhaps understand what the literature is saying about your topic.

How Can Matrices Be Combined and Why Should They Be?

The Matrix Method has been described as the activity by one person who is reviewing the literature on a specific topic. This method can be extended to use by two or more people with two or more topics. Here is an example. Suppose a clinical outcomes research group in a large, managed care organization needed to review the literature about a medical device that became available on the market 10 years ago. The goal of this team was to understand what the research has to say about the clinical effectiveness of the medical device for use by patients. The organization's clinical board was interested in possibly recommending the device to clinicians in its network. The research team consisted of a physician, nurse practitioner, biostatistician, epidemiologist, and consumer advocate. All were accomplished in the use of the Matrix Method; RefWorks, which was their organization's reference management software; and a variety of electronic bibliographic databases such as MEDLINE and CINAHL. Should one of these team members review the literature and summarize the results for the others? What would be the benefit if they all reviewed the literature? If all participated in the review, how would they divide up the work?

The group decided that each team member would review all of the literature because they all needed to be at the same level of understanding of research about the device. They began by discussing the purpose of the review, then each would apply the Matrix Method separately and compare their progress at four stages: (1) selection of articles, (2) creation of the column topics, (3) completion of the Review Matrix, and (4) draft of the synthesis. They agreed at the beginning that each reviewer would have a different focus: the physician would concentrate on clinical outcomes and medical factors related to its use, the nurse practitioner would focus on patient factors that contributed to success or failure of the device; the biostatistician would be responsible for evaluating the methods and statistical procedures and explaining the statistical outcomes to the group; the epidemiologist would be concerned about population findings about use in different settings (home, community, nursing home), in different geographic areas, and under other conditions in which the device was used; and the consumer advocate would focus on patient reactions and evaluations about ease of use in everyday life. Team members set about the task separately in identifying articles and creating column topics.

(Continues)

EXHIBIT 7-1 FAQs About Getting the Most Out of the Matrix Method (*Continued*)

The reason the team members compared their results at four points was to standardize the review. The final selection of articles to be reviewed were those collected by all team members. They realized that some articles might not be relevant to their focus, but all team members would have to critically analyze each article by its purpose, methods, and relevance to the general purpose. This meant that when one team member described a study, they all were familiar with the content. The discussion of the column topics also reflected all of their input. They used a decision rule of agreeing on general topics such as purpose, methods, description of data collection instruments, methodological design, and statistical procedures.

Then each had a section specific to his or her own focus. Everybody had a final column in which they could record their impression of the study. Each completed the Review Matrix separately. They went over the results of these review matrices in a discussion section and agreed on the outline and content of the synthesis. Each drafted the synthesis for his or her own focus. The result was a document that reflected all of their investments of time and effort, their expertise, and their focus, and they agreed on the recommendations to the board.

In another example, a class of students took a similar approach when they divided up into teams of five and used the Matrix Method to review the same topic but worked separately until they came together to prepare the synthesis based on their independently prepared review matrices.

What Is Plagiarism?

Plagiarism is claiming the work of others as your own. Books, articles, and websites have discussed this problem at length. The focus here is to describe how to avoid it in the context of the Matrix Method. Always put quotation marks around any material you copy directly from a source document and record the citation at the end of the quote. When you are preparing the synthesis of the review of the literature, describe the quoted material in your own words. It is still necessary to show where the ideas (written in your own words) came from (i.e., always cite your sources).

Caroline's Quest: Building Her Own Library of Master Folders

In addition to working on her master's thesis, Caroline also had several term papers to write for her other courses. In her developmental psychology course, Caroline reviewed the literature on differences in self-esteem between male and female adolescents. Some of the research articles she included in that review were the same papers she had included in her thesis.

Caroline wanted to create an electronic reprint file that she could maintain during and after her graduate school program. Professor Dickerson suggested that she set up a reprint filing system around a library of Master Folders with a Documents Folder in each. Because she planned to have multiple Master Folders, she assigned the same label to each of the four folders within each Master Folder. For example, the Self-Esteem Master Folder included the Self-Esteem Paper Trail Folder, the Self-Esteem Documents Folder, the Self-Esteem Review Matrix Folder, and the Self-Esteem Synthesis Folder. For her thesis literature review she created the Adolescent Smoking Master Folder, which included the following four folders: Adolescent Smoking Paper Trail Folder, Adolescent Smoking Documents Folder, Adolescent Smoking Review Matrix Folder, and Adolescent Smoking Synthesis Folder.

Caroline used the self-esteem and smoking article both in the paper she wrote for the course on adolescent development and in her thesis. The paper was filed only once, however, in the Self-Esteem Documents Folder, because it was created before she began reviewing the literature for her thesis. By using the Matrix Indexing System, Caroline was able to keep track of whether she had a copy of an article and where each was filed. She could also just make a copy of the paper from the Adolescent Smoking Documents Folder and put that copy in the Self-Esteem Documents Folder. The choice was hers.

Over the 2 years of her graduate program, Caroline accumulated six Master Folders, including one on research methods and another on public health interventions. Depending on which subject each Master Folder covered, she included notes from national meetings and government reports. Some of these additions were included after the literature review was completed. These Master Folders were stored in her Master Folders library, a library that grew over the years as she added new articles and documents from her work. An important part of maintaining that library was keeping an up-to-date record of the materials she had and where they were stored. Thus, an integral part of creating and using a Master Folders library is its integration with the Matrix Indexing System.

REFERENCE

1. Garrard J, Choudary V, Groom H, et al. Organizational change in management of hepatitis C: evaluation of a CME program. *J Contin Educ Health Prof.* 2006;26(2);145-160.

CHAPTER 8

The Matrix Indexing System

The Matrix Indexing System described in this chapter consists of merging information from three different sources: electronic bibliographic databases, reference management software, and the Source Documents Subfolders located in one or more Master Folders. The topics covered in this chapter are as follows:

- What Is the Matrix Indexing System?
- How to Set Up a Matrix Indexing System
- How to Expand the Source Documents Subfolder
- How to Efficiently Update a Synthesis
- Caroline's Quest: Using the Matrix Indexing System

WHAT IS THE MATRIX INDEXING SYSTEM?

How do you create a system for organizing materials across multiple reviews of the literature over time as you add new source documents and share them with colleagues or associates? The Matrix Indexing System was developed for just these purposes. It is a plan for organizing your references and documents and managing this information on an ongoing basis. This indexing system can be useful throughout a professional career, whether you begin using it as a student or later in your career.

The Matrix Indexing System consists of these activities:

- Merging information from three sources: (1) an electronic bibliographic database, such as MEDLINE; (2) reference management software, such as RefWorks, EndNote, or ProCite; and (3) the Source Documents Subfolder (located in the Documents Folder in your Master Folder)

- Expanding the Source Documents Subfolder in your Master Folder
- Updating a synthesis of the review of the literature

Advantages of the Matrix Indexing System

If you set up your initial review of the literature using the Matrix Method, you already have a start on the Matrix Indexing System. However, the indexing system differs from the Matrix Method. The Matrix Method is a strategy for acquiring, analyzing, and writing a synthesis of a review of the scientific literature. In contrast, the Matrix Indexing System provides a way of coping with all the information and documents that you use or create as a result of a review of the literature. In other words, the Matrix Indexing System gives you a way to create a manageable system in the afterlife of each review of the literature. This chapter explains how to create and use the Matrix Indexing System.

HOW TO SET UP A MATRIX INDEXING SYSTEM

You need four tools to create a Matrix Indexing System: electronic bibliographic databases, reference management software, source documents downloaded and stored chronologically in the Source Documents Subfolder (located in the Documents Folder), and location labels.

Electronic Bibliographic Databases

From your own computer, you must be able to access one or more of the electronic bibliographic databases, such as MEDLINE, CINAHL, or others. A dozen or more electronic bibliographic databases are available to health sciences professionals, and more are being created at a rapid rate. MEDLINE is the oldest and largest of these databases in the health sciences. Check with the reference librarian at a biomedical library about new databases that have come online in recent months. In this context, the term *index* is used interchangeably with *database*.

An effort is under way by the National Science Foundation to encourage the development and use of electronic libraries. Their availability over the coming years might offer additional resources to professionals in the health sciences. Check out further information on the National Library of Medicine website at http://gateway.nlm.nih.gov/gw/Cmd/about.jsp.

In describing the role of an electronic bibliographic database in the Matrix Indexing System, MEDLINE is used as the example, although this indexing system applies to many other databases and probably to those that have not yet become available.

Reference Management Software

You need to purchase and install reference management software, such as End-Note or ProCite, for your own computer. If your institution has a subscription to the web-based product, RefWorks, you can set up your own free database of references. Contact your institution's librarian to find out more about this option. Currently all of these packages (EndNote, ProCite, and RefWorks) have the capability to download information from an electronic bibliographic database to users' computers.

Further information about EndNote can be found at http://www.endnote .com; information on ProCite is at http://www.procite.com; and details about RefWorks can be found at http://www.refworks.com. You only need one of these reference management software packages. In choosing one, ask yourself whether you can use it over a long period of time. For example, if you are interested in RefWorks because your university library has a site license and offers it free to students over the Internet, find out from the librarian what the rules are for continuing to use RefWorks after you graduate or leave the university. You may have to pay a monthly fee for continued use, but it may be worth the cost.

Software packages designed to format references in research papers and reports have been available for approximately 15–20 years, and they can be used with a variety of computer platforms, such as Mac, PC, and Unix. Reference management software is also known as bibliographic management or citation management software.

Organizing and Printing References Using Reference Management Software

You can organize references to scientific papers, books, and other source documents cited in scientific or other academic publications and arrange them in the references section of a scientific paper according to your choice of bibliographic style—this is the reference management part of these software packages. The software packages offer numerous bibliographic styles to choose from, including American Psychological Association, American Medical Association, the Vancouver style used by many medical journals, Modern Language Association of America, Nature, Proceedings of the National Academy of Science, and the Turabian Reference List style based on the book *A Manual for Writers of Term Papers, Theses, and Dissertations*.[1]

In preparing a manuscript to be submitted to a journal or for a report or thesis, there is an enormous savings in time and effort in being able to switch from one bibliographic style, such as the AMA style for the *Journal of the American Medical Association* (*JAMA*) in the medical field, to another style, such as the

APA style for *American Psychologist*. This capability alone is reason enough to put a reference management software package on your computer. Over time, however, these packages have developed additional features that are now put to use in the Matrix Indexing System.

Downloading References and Abstracts Using Reference Management Software

Reference management software packages provide a link between electronic bibliographic databases, located in places like a biomedical library or on the Internet, and a reference library on your own computer. Reference management software such as EndNote or RefWorks uses the term *reference library*. In the Matrix Method, this is the same as the Source Documents Subfolder. With the reference management software, you can download references, including abstracts of journal articles, directly from electronic databases such as MEDLINE to your computer, which means you do not have to retype or paste the information—the software does it for you. If you have difficulty downloading references and abstracts from your library, check with a reference librarian for special instructions. Often university-based libraries conduct tutorials about how to use reference management software packages; check to see whether such classes are available at your library.

Source Documents Subfolder = Your Reference Library

You can create and maintain one or more user-specified reference libraries (Source Documents Subfolders) on your computer—the software sets them up for you. Read the manual for the software package you are using.

You can sort references in your Source Documents Subfolder by author, year of publication, journal, topic, or any other category you specify. Most reference management programs also have a search capability that helps you find articles within the references you have stored using whatever terms you choose. For example, you can find all the articles in your own ProCite library that mention the words *randomized clinical trial.*

There is also flexibility about where you will search in your Source Documents Subfolder. For example, you can direct the search to include the document title, the abstract, and notes you have written about the article. This is a real advantage because the likelihood of finding a source document will be increased if you include a search of the abstract. This search feature is a good reason for always downloading an abstract from the electronic bibliographic database rather than restricting yourself to just the author's name, article title, and journal issue. The manual for the software package explains how to do this. (Note, this manual often can be found online; check with your reference librarian for where the manual is for the software package you are using.)

In addition to searching each reference in the information downloaded from the electronic bibliographic database into your own Source Documents Subfolder, you can also create your own key words or labels, store them in a particular part of the reference file, and then search on those labels. Some of the programs have set aside sections just for this purpose. For example, three such sections provided in EndNote are labels, key words, and notes. You have to decide which section you consistently will use for storing your location label for each article. These two features, storing a key word in a specific location and the search capability, are especially helpful for using a standard list of location labels to keep track of where your source documents can be found.

Location Labels for Master Folders

Location labels describe where you keep your reprints or other source documents. These location labels provide a link between the references in your reference management software and the reprints in the Source Documents Subfolders in one or more Master Folders. In creating a standard list of location labels, the most efficient strategy is to make this list before you do a review of the literature or accumulate reprints in the Source Documents Subfolder. This means that you will need to use the reference management software package from the beginning. For example, at the initial stage of the review of the literature, as you search the electronic databases for relevant papers in research journals, you can download the references and their corresponding abstracts of interesting papers into your Source Documents Subfolder. By the time you have completed the review of the literature, you will probably have a large set of references in your Source Documents Subfolder, only some of which have corresponding reprints.

Create a list of location labels by tagging each reference in your Source Documents Subfolder. Use a standard label for the name of the three Name of Master Folders. For example, suppose that you have three Master Folders with related content: one on antidepressants, another on depression, and a third on research methods in psychiatry. Use a location label for each of the downloaded copies of journal articles. The location label for the first Master Folder would be Psych—Antidepressants; the second would be labeled Psych—Depression; and the third would be labeled Psych—Research Methods. By always putting these labels in a specific location in the reference file, such as the notes section or the label section, or whatever category is available in the computer package you use, you can search these categories for specific key words to find where you stored any reprint you have in your Master Folders. An example of adding this tag to the label section of a reference in EndNote is shown in **Exhibit 8-1**.

EXHIBIT 8-1 Example of a Standard Label for a Fictional Paper Located in the Source Documents Subfolder of the Psych—Depression Master Folder

---

Author
Smith, Harriet
Year
1997
Title
Differences between psychotherapy and tricyclic antidepressants in the treatment of depression
Journal
Journal of Treatment
Volume
67
Issue
15
Pages
1203–1208
Label
Psych—Depression
Key Words
depression, antidepressants, psychotherapy
Abstract (Your Own Summary)
This was a randomized, clinical trial of psychotherapy and tricyclic antidepressants. 100 female outpatients in a managed care organization were evaluated weekly on a prepost basis. Study period was 1 year and assessment with the . . .
Notes
Excellent methodological design with sufficient numbers of subjects ranging in age from 21 to 64 years. Results show that . . .

Location Labels for Materials Not Stored in the Source Documents Subfolder

You may not have a downloaded copy of all the documents that you abstracted in your review matrix. Some documents may be in the form of books or chapters or reports that are available in your own library. Other source documents may be located elsewhere, such as those in a department library or a regional library. These materials may be too long to be photocopied, despite their usefulness in your review of the literature. For example, a chapter in a standard statistics book might be the key reference that describes an important analytical technique.

Location labels can help you to remember what these references are and where they are located. Keep track of these references by creating a set of labels analogous to the Psych—Master Folder label. For example, instead of using the name of a Master Folder in the label, you might choose another standard set of words, such as Reprint—Own Library or Reprint—Biomedical Library. Thus, a label such as Reprint—Own Library for the statistics book located on the shelf in your office might be the standard label that you use to find the chapter with the analytical technique. The word *reprint* is a useful common tag because it enables you to sort all references on that word alone and find the documents quickly and efficiently.

How the Elements Are Linked

Location labels, together with reference management software, are the keys to managing an overwhelming amount of detail about PDF files, printed documents, or other materials accumulated in a literature review. You might store such a list in a specific section in the Paper Trail Folder. If nothing else, tape a copy of your list of location labels to the back of your office door. The point is to create and use location labels as part of the Matrix Indexing System to manage the materials you accumulate, use intensively, and then forget about them until you need to access them quickly at a later date.

An illustration of how the different elements of a Matrix Indexing System are linked by the reference management software and the location labels is summarized in **Figure 8-1**. Specifically, references and abstracts of journal articles and other materials are downloaded from an electronic bibliographic database, such as MEDLINE, into your Source Documents Subfolder on your computer using reference management software such as RefWorks. Using the same reference management software, you create a standard list of location labels and tag each reference in your Source Documents Subfolder with its location. The advantage

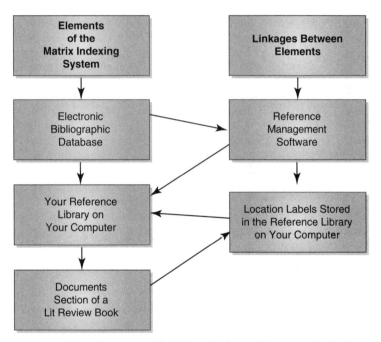

FIGURE 8-1 How elements in the Matrix Indexing System are linked together.

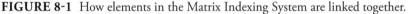

of storing all your reprints chronologically in a Source Documents Subfolder and then keeping track of the references in your reference library using location labels is that you will be able to find these materials when you need them. Thus, you create an organized storage and filing system for your reprints, rather than a random collection of articles that you cannot access because you cannot remember what is there or how to locate the materials you need.

HOW TO EXPAND THE SOURCE DOCUMENTS SUBFOLDER

As the number of reprints you download increases, you may face the problem of information overload. One way to manage this problem is to create a new Master Folder with another title. For example, suppose your initial literature review was on hepatitis C and you have downloaded 100 PDFs on this topic in your Source Documents Subfolder. Over the years, your focus has become more detailed, and you are now interested in reviewing the literature on outcomes associated with specific treatments of this disease. You might consider starting a new Master

Folder (which you could call Hep C Tx Outcomes Master Folder) and begin to download PDFs into your Source Documents Subfolder on this topic.

As you create and use these Master Folders, you might want to truncate the names to something manageable, such as Hep C Outcomes Master Folder and the corresponding Hep C Outcomes Paper Trail Folder, the Hep C Outcomes Documents Folder and so forth for the remaining folders.

It is useful to always include a standard set of names for your folders so you can perform a quick and reliable search of your desktop for information. For example, using the search term, Master Folder, could produce all of the Master Folders you have created for any literature review.

HOW TO EFFICIENTLY UPDATE A SYNTHESIS

If you review the literature on a topic once and never look at those source documents or return to that topic again, then you can skip this section. If, however, you need to evaluate new information or consider source documents added since the original review on the same subject, you need a strategy for updating your review of the literature. One of the simplest ways to do this is to abstract the source documents you have added since the last review and bring the review matrix and the synthesis up to date.

A typical scenario for an experienced scientist is when an extensive review of the literature is prepared as part of a grant proposal, and the Master Folder is set aside during the period when the grant is reviewed. After the grant is awarded, the research begins, with new references identified and new source documents added in the Source Documents Subfolder as they become available. Later, in preparing scientific papers about the results of the study, another thorough review of the literature is needed, probably with a more specific focus than for the grant proposal. The same Master Folder can be used for these purposes: generation of the initial literature review for the proposal, creation and use of a Source Documents Subfolder for storing and adding reprints of research papers over time, an update of the Review Matrix, and preparation of a new Synthesis Folder for the literature review for the manuscript describing the results of a completed study. Over the same period of time, from grant proposal to publication of research results, this Master Folder has kept pace with the researcher.

In general, updating a review of the literature is more efficient, more thorough, and quicker if the materials are organized and updated as you go along. Materials such as a reference library, which might be available on a server that can be accessed by all members of a research team, and the Master Folder, which might be stored in a central location for the same team, are invaluable resources that will help advance the research effort.

Caroline's Quest: Using the Matrix Indexing System

In her review of the literature, Caroline was interested in exploring the possibility of a link between smoking by teenage girls and depression. As an initial step, she searched for a review article on depression. The process she used illustrates the Matrix Indexing System, from identifying the paper in the electronic bibliographic database, to downloading the abstract with her reference management software, to making a note that she had a copy of the article in the Source Documents Subfolder in a Master Folder.

Caroline began by logging on to PubMed through the university library on her computer. She searched for a review article that she had identified earlier, one by Leon and colleagues.[2] She downloaded the reference and abstract to her computer. Using EndNote, which was the reference management software Caroline had on her computer, she imported the reference and abstract into her Source Documents Subfolder, which she had titled Teenagers & Smoking References.

In the standard EndNote abstract form, she also wrote a note that she had a reprint of the entire article stored in the Source Documents Subfolder within her Depression Master Folder located in the Master Folder library.

Several days later Caroline met with Professor Dickerson to discuss her progress. By this time she had a large file of reprints and was having trouble keeping track of them all. She asked, "What do you do when there are too many reprints? I can't create more and more Source Documents Subfolders."

"Well," he told her, "when that happens, you might think about organizing them by decade of publication." He pointed to the screen of his own computer, "For example, the 109 reprints I have on depression are located in three Source Documents Subfolders in the Depression Master Folder, which I've separated chronologically by publication in 1980–1989, 1990–1994, and 1995–present. They are labeled Depression (1980–89) Source Documents, Depression (1990–94) Source Documents, and Depression (1995–present) Source Documents. Because they are indexed by year of publication, neither my students nor I have any problem finding a specific reprint."

Caroline made a note of Professor Dickerson's strategy for handling too many reprints and then talked about her use of the Matrix Indexing System. "I guess this system could be used with any kind of literature review," she reflected, "whether or not it is of the scientific literature."

Professor Dickerson described how a colleague who was an author of a series of books on gardening used the Matrix Indexing System for keeping track of his notes, gardening catalogs, and reprints from popular magazines about gardening tips. "It really is a sensible way of organizing a lot of material," he agreed.

REFERENCES

1. Turabian KL. *A Manual for Writers of Term Papers, Theses, and Dissertations*. 6th ed. Chicago, IL: University of Chicago Press; 1996.
2. Leon AC, Klerman GL, Wickramaratne P. Continuing female predominance in depressive illness. *Am J Public Health*. 1993;83:754-757.

CHAPTER 9

Matrix Applications by Health Sciences Professionals

The purpose of this chapter is to describe examples of how the Matrix Method and the Matrix Indexing System can be used in some of the more advanced research and development activities in the health sciences. The following examples are included in this chapter:

- What Are Matrix Applications?
- How to Use Matrix Applications in a Research Project
- How to Use Matrix Applications in a Meta-Analysis
- How to Use Matrix Applications in Practice Guidelines
- How to Use Matrix Applications in Evidence-Based Medicine
- Caroline's Quest: Matrix Applications in Nonscientific Settings

WHAT ARE MATRIX APPLICATIONS?

A matrix application is the use of the concepts and procedures of the Matrix Method, the Matrix Indexing System, or both.

The Matrix Method is a plan for gathering materials to be included in a review of the literature, systematically analyzing the information, writing a synthesis, and organizing and filing documents, notes, and other materials in one of four folders (Paper Trail Folder, Documents Folder, Review Matrix Folder, or Synthesis Folder) in a Master Folder during and after the review.

The Matrix Indexing System is a set of procedures for bringing together information from three sources: (1) one or more electronic bibliographic databases such as MEDLINE or CINAHL; (2) reference management software, such as RefWorks, EndNote, or ProCite; and (3) copies of scientific papers and other materials stored in the Source Documents Subfolder (located in the Documents Folder in the Master Folder).

Advantages of Matrix Applications

Used either separately or together, the Matrix Method and the Matrix Indexing System offer an efficient strategy that can be used throughout the career of a health sciences professional in a variety of settings, including the following:

- Academia
- Research and evaluation consulting firms
- Clinical settings, such as public hospitals, private practices or facilities, or managed care organizations
- City, county, and state departments of health and public health
- Government and health policy organizations responsible for policy analysis or development of health legislation and regulations
- Research and development departments in the private sector or health-related industries, such as pharmaceutical or medical electronics companies
- Consumer health information organizations, such as those that produce science magazines and newsletters, patient information brochures for managed care organizations or hospitals, and health and science sections of daily newspapers

Matrix applications can be used interactively by a group of people. For example, in setting up a matrix indexing system for use by a group, the Source Documents Subfolder created with reference management software, such as EndNote or RefWorks, could be maintained on a server or in a cloud that is accessible to all members of the group. Reprints of the research papers and other scientific articles filed chronologically in the Source Documents Subfolder could be maintained in the same central location. A system for adding new source documents and accessing them could be developed among members of the team. (A website for EndNote can be found at this website: http://endnote.com; and for RefWorks in academic settings at this website: http://www.proquest.com/libraries/academic/.)

Whether used by an individual or a group, the Matrix Method and the Matrix Indexing System offer a versatile and useful strategy for conducting a review of the literature and maintaining a library of reprints in a variety of settings. This is a cost-effective and time-efficient strategy for busy health sciences professionals. Examples of how this strategy can be used in the context of different kinds of activities are described in the remainder of this chapter.

The example used in Caroline's Quest at the end of this chapter departs from the traditional scientific setting and describes how matrix applications can be modified and used to prepare background information for a lay audience. Whether the author's intent is to communicate research findings to other scientists or to describe the latest breakthrough in medicine to readers of a daily newspaper, matrix applications can be used to organize the writer's reprints, notes, and thoughts.

HOW TO USE MATRIX APPLICATIONS IN A RESEARCH PROJECT

A typical research project has several stages of development, from conception of the idea to publication of the final results. These stages may vary depending on the researcher, the reason for doing the project, and the goals of the research. In an academic setting, research projects in the health sciences generally follow three stages: (1) preparation of a proposal describing the hypothesis and methods for carrying out the study (sometimes this is a grant proposal, which is a request for funding of the study), (2) implementation of the project after approval or funding has been obtained, and (3) preparation of the written reports and papers to be submitted for publication in peer-reviewed journals, a stage that often transitions between the research project itself and after the project has been completed.

The Matrix Method and the Matrix Indexing System can be used to access, analyze, and manage references, reprints, and reviews of the literature at each of these stages in the research process. The application of these tools can also have a cumulative advantage because the information and the files acquired at each stage build on those gathered at the previous stage.

For example, preparing a grant proposal is rarely a linear activity that progresses in lockstep from the generation of an idea, to reviewing the literature, to planning the methodology, to writing the proposal. In reality, these activities occur more or less simultaneously. Although each of these tasks may dominate the researchers' time and attention at any point in the process, there is often the need to recheck the literature in the midst of planning the methodology or to rethink the research questions as plans for the proposed analysis are being finalized.

Most experienced researchers have a working knowledge of the research literature as they think about ideas for a new study for months or even years. As these thoughts germinate, additional possibilities for studies may be suggested in publications, presentations at scientific meetings, or in discussions with colleagues. Additional publications, such as newly published journal articles, can be stored in a Source Documents Subfolder within a Master Folder. A chronological list of the reprints can be kept in the Source Documents Subfolder on the scientist's computer.

When ideas for a research study begin to take shape, a more intensive effort may be mounted to review the literature systematically, especially on topics tangentially related to the research idea or to methodological approaches that might be applicable. At this point, a Review Matrix can be set up, the choice of column topics made, and the research literature abstracted.

Finally, when the grant proposal or other research document is written, tracking down specific references or locating studies in areas where there appear to be gaps in the knowledge base will intensify. This is the point when a synthesis is written, based on the literature abstracted in the Review Matrix.

By developing and maintaining a Matrix Indexing System from the mulling-over period to its use in the completion of a Review Matrix, researchers can accumulate the materials they need to abstract the literature and write a concise synthesis. Often there is a strict limitation on the number of pages in a grant proposal. The literature review, which is one small part of the proposal, has to be accurate, thorough, and concise. For example, most National Institutes of Health grant proposals have a strict page limit, of which the literature review is a very small part. Therefore, previous knowledge about the topic has to be distilled and thoroughly accurate. The Review Matrix is a useful tool in this distillation process. Writing a Synthesis is an even more refined tool.

After the research project is funded, the researcher will continue to read the scientific literature and download new publications to the Source Documents Subfolder, using reference management software such as RefWorks to maintain an up-to-date reprint file of the relevant studies. Later, when the project has progressed to the preparation of scientific papers or reports, health scientists with an up-to-date Source Documents Subfolder in their Master Folder are in a good position to update the Review Matrix of previously abstracted papers and write a more current synthesis that includes the recently added research papers.

HOW TO USE MATRIX APPLICATIONS IN A META-ANALYSIS

A meta-analysis consists of the statistical evaluation of multiple research studies or clinical trials on a specific topic. The procedures for a meta-analysis require that a study protocol be clearly specified. The first task is to describe the purpose, the methodology, and especially the criteria for selecting studies. Next, the studies to be analyzed must be selected and reviewed. Finally, the statistical procedures for summarizing the results are applied to the set of studies included in the analysis.

The Matrix Method provides a structure for carrying out the first two stages of a meta-analysis. For example, the criteria for the kinds of studies to be gathered and a complete record of how the literature was searched can be documented in the Paper Trail Folder located in the Master Folder. This is the first draft of the authors' adaptation of the PRISMA Flowchart[1] which might be stored in either the Paper Trail Folder or in the Documents Folder. After the studies for the meta-analysis are selected, they can be assembled and filed chronologically in the Source Documents Subfolder. Then the critical elements of purpose and research methodology can be abstracted in a Review Matrix. The information needed for the statistical analysis can also be included as column topics in the Review Matrix.

The advantage of using the Matrix Method becomes even more apparent if the meta-analysis is being done by two or more people. Often a large number of scientific papers have to be reviewed before a final decision is made about which studies meet the criteria. This task could be assigned to multiple people who use a Review Matrix with the same set of column topics. Then the final selection of the studies to be included in the meta-analysis could be based on the information abstracted in their review matrices.

The primary emphasis in a meta-analysis is on the statistical summary of empirical studies and the interpretation of those results; however, these end points could be compromised by the ways in which the tasks of selecting and reviewing the basic materials—the studies to be analyzed—are carried out. The Matrix Method and the Matrix Indexing System provide an additional level of organization and efficiency in rigorously accomplishing those fundamental tasks for a meta-analysis.

Although this guide is tailored largely to graduate students for use in an academic setting, the Matrix Method and the Matrix Indexing System are applicable to research in other arenas as well. The following two sections outline the use of matrix applications for developing clinical practice guidelines and for performing research for evidence-based medicine.

HOW TO USE MATRIX APPLICATIONS IN PRACTICE GUIDELINES

Practice guidelines give healthcare providers, such as physicians, nurses, and allied health professionals, sound strategies for delivering the best possible health care based on the scientific literature. Although practice guidelines initially were created by nationally based teams of healthcare professionals under the sponsorship of organizations such as the Agency for Healthcare Research and Quality, recently such development has shifted to more local or regional groups made up of clinicians within healthcare organizations, reimbursement companies, and even small practice groups.

The fundamental concept in developing a clinical practice guideline is to create a set of best practices for diagnosing, treating, managing, and preventing a clinical condition based on the scientific literature. A review of the literature is a necessary first step, and matrix applications can be an integral part of this phase in the development of a practice guideline.

Consider, for example, a team of clinicians in an outpatient clinic consisting of a pediatric nurse practitioner, a pediatrician, and a telephone triage or intake nurse who work together to develop a practice guideline on otitis media (middle ear infection) in young children. After agreeing on the definition of the condition and the criteria for the guideline, they divide the task of reviewing the literature based on the process and the structure of the Matrix Method.

The intake nurse reviews the literature on symptoms of the condition. The pediatrician focuses on current research on treatment and clinical management, and the nurse practitioner concentrates on studies about prevention of otitis media at the individual and community levels. By coordinating their efforts through the use of a single Master Folder, the task is accomplished in less time than it would take an individual. For example, they meet to agree on the criteria for the search, maintain a log of the strategies they used and the electronic databases and other sources they consulted, and generate an ongoing list of key words. This information is recorded in the Paper Trail Folder, which is stored in a central location that they all can access (e.g., in the cloud). The documents they gather, including reprints of studies, examples of guidelines from other groups, and papers from secondary and tertiary sources such as the Cochrane Library, are filed in the Source Documents Subfolder. Later in the process, they make a joint decision about the column topics to be included in a Review Matrix.

In abstracting the documents in the Review Matrix, the strategy this team chose was to have the three members read all of the documents, with each team member abstracting a subset of the column topics. For example, the physician abstracted all of the documents for column topics concerned with treatment and management, and the nurse practitioner abstracted the same set of articles on recognition of symptoms. By the time the guideline was ready to be written, all of the team members were thoroughly versed in the scientific literature.

In this example, the column topics might include methodological issues, but the focus was on the major subheadings of the guideline, such as symptom recognition, diagnosis, treatment, management, and prevention. The purpose of the guideline will dictate the choice of column topics for the Review Matrix.

The Matrix Indexing System would also be an asset in preparing a clinical guideline as the literature is being reviewed and then later in updating the guideline. For example, once a year a member of the original team uses the same search strategy with the same electronic bibliographic databases, such as MEDLINE and CINAHL, to identify new studies on the same topic. During the same period of time, team members or any of the other practitioners in the outpatient clinic add scientific papers or other materials to the Source Documents Subfolder within the Otitis Media Master Folder located on the server for the office. One person in the clinic is responsible for coordinating all Master Folders on a variety of clinical topics of interest to the clinicians.

Matrix applications will not accomplish all of the tasks needed to develop clinical practice guidelines, but they can provide an efficient process and a well-defined structure for accomplishing the task. Matrix applications can also be especially useful when a team of healthcare professionals must coordinate their efforts to produce a single product in the form of a guideline for the care of patients with a specific condition.

HOW TO USE MATRIX APPLICATIONS IN EVIDENCE-BASED MEDICINE

Evidence-based medicine is as much a philosophy about the importance of using current research findings as a basis for clinical decisions as it is a series of well-defined users' guides for understanding how to read and interpret the literature. There are 32 users' guides published in JAMA, and more are expected in the future.[2-33] The Matrix Method and the Matrix Indexing System are consistent with the principles of evidence-based medicine and can provide a structure and process for implementing this approach.

Consider, for example, a nurse practitioner in a diabetes clinic who wants to develop an outpatient program on diet and exercise for her older patients that would emphasize improvement in their quality of life. She begins by reading the users' guide published in the 1997 issue of the *Journal of the American Medical Association* (*JAMA*) on how to use articles about health-related quality of life.[18] After she understands the principles of this type of research described in that users' guide, she begins her search of the current literature. She also stores a copy of the users' in the Source Documents Subfolder (in the Documents Folder) in order to have it handy.

Using the principles of the Matrix Method, she looks up the users' guide on MEDLINE and records the medical subject headings, some of which include quality of life, quality-adjusted life years, and patient care planning. The medical subject headings go in a list she creates in the Key Words Subfolder, as described in Chapter 3. She then searches MEDLINE for this type of article in combination with key words describing the condition, such as diabetes, diet, and exercise. She also examines the list of references at the end of the users' guide on health-related quality of life to identify studies that might be related to her topic of interest.

Although her focus is on the quality of life of older people, she realizes that research in this area is relatively recent and might not have included people older than 65 years old. For that reason, she does not limit her MEDLINE search by age of subjects. She keeps notes in the Paper Trail Folder on the key words, procedures, and search strategies she used.

After she reviews the references and abstracts of the studies online, she downloads the reprints from MEDLINE and CINAHL into a Source Documents Subfolder on her computer using EndNote. Next she uses MEDLINE to search for specific articles and downloads those that are most relevant to her topic. In deciding which column topics to use in setting up the Review Matrix, the nurse practitioner again consults the users' guide on health-related quality of life. She includes as column topics some of the issues raised in that article, such as whether the research studies measured aspects of patients' lives that the patients themselves considered important and characteristics of the data collection instruments, especially the validity of the questionnaire. In general, the users' guide helps the nurse practitioner think about the kinds of issues that she needs to consider in her own review of the literature.

After she abstracts the research studies in the Review Matrix, the nurse practitioner writes a brief synthesis of the literature as a basis for deciding which instrument to use in measuring health-related quality of life in her clinical practice. In the process of identifying research studies from MEDLINE and CINAHL, she creates a Source Documents Subfolder on health-related quality of life and uses a location label in each reference in the Source Documents Subfolder located in her Quality of Life Master Folder.

Throughout this process of identifying keywords, finding source documents, creating a Review Matrix and abstracting the relevant source documents, the nurse practitioner records the numbers of documents at each stage of the review process and fills in the PRISMA Flowchart[1] so she can document her search. The completed PRISMA Flowchart becomes part of the synthesis she writes that becomes part of her narrative review of the literature.

Caroline's Quest: Matrix Applications in Nonscientific Settings

One of the requirements of Caroline's master's degree program is a 3-month internship in the community. Caroline was interested in applying what she had learned in her public health courses to help people in the community understand and use current research findings to improve their own health. She therefore chose to do her internship with a science writer for a local city newspaper. Caroline's first assignment was to do background research for a three-part series of articles to be published in the newspaper on how to prevent injuries to children in day care centers.

The newspaper's health reporter, who was responsible for the final writing of the series of articles, was Caroline's mentor for the internship. Together they developed an outline that Caroline would follow to gather information needed for writing the articles. The topics for the three articles were (1) a description of the kinds of injuries to children in day care settings and what their causes were, (2) how such injuries can be prevented, and (3) a checklist for parents to use as they determined whether a day care center gave sufficient attention to prevention of injuries to children.

Caroline began by searching some of the major electronic bibliographic databases, including MEDLINE from 1985 to the present, Current Contents from 1994 to the present, and CINAHL from 1982 to the present. She found three research studies from these sources.[34–36] She downloaded each of these papers into her Source Documents Subfolder.

Next, Caroline called the state health department and talked to the director of the office responsible for licensing day care centers about the reporting of day care injuries. She recorded her notes on a standard interview form that she had created, shown in **Exhibit 9-1**. Caroline also obtained a copy of the statistics for fatal and nonfatal injuries to children in day care over the past 5 years. She made a PDF copy of her notes and stored it in her Paper Trail Folder.

Caroline's reporter mentor looked over the information Caroline had collected and advised her to do some telephone interviews with experts in the field.

EXHIBIT 9-1 Caroline's Interview Form

Date _____ Time _____

Person Interviewed _____

Job Title and Department of Person Interviewed _____

Company/Organization _____

Telephone _____ Fax _____

E-mail _____

Interview Topic _____

Notes and Quotes _____

_____

_____

_____

Additional Contacts or Leads Suggested _____

_____

_____

"How do I locate the experts?" Caroline asked. "Maybe I could try to call the authors of the research articles?" she looked inquisitively at the reporter.

Her mentor smiled, "Yes, but a quicker way to solve that problem would be to contact the people at ProfNet and find out whether there are any local experts with information that would be of interest to our readers."

"What's ProfNet?" Caroline asked.

"It's an Internet service staffed by public relations experts at colleges and universities across the country that provides journalists and authors with leads on expert sources from more than 4,000 colleges, universities, think tanks, national laboratories, hospitals, nonprofit organizations, corporations, and public relations agencies. Our newspaper has a subscription to this service. Look up their website; I'll send you the link. The ProfNet section you should access for this series of articles is Health/Medicine." The mentor sent her a link to ProfNet: http://www.prnewswire.com/profnet/profnet-journalists/.

As a result of her inquiries on ProfNet, Caroline contacted professors at two nearby universities and a staff person at a nonprofit organization for prevention of childhood injuries. She recorded her notes from each interview on her standardized interview form.

During the first week of her internship, Caroline also searched other sites on the Internet, such as some of the leading newspapers, state and federal agencies responsible for regulation of day care centers, and local and statewide associations of licensed day care providers. From these sources she identified parents, day care providers, and community leaders who were willing to be interviewed. She called several people in each of these categories.

Caroline used the Matrix Method to organize the information she collected for the newspaper assignment. First, she created a Master Folder with the usual four folders: Paper Trail, Documents, Review Matrix, and Synthesis. In the Paper Trail Folder, she documented her search activities and added a subsection on interviews where she kept a list of interviewees by date and other people they suggested that she contact. This list was actually a record of her use of the snowball technique applied to people, rather than references, as Professor Dickerson had initially taught her.

Caroline modified the standard approach of the Matrix Method to meet her needs in this nonscientific setting. First, she expanded the Documents Folder within the Master Folder by adding three subfolders: Research Studies, Interviews, and Statistics. After she had collected sufficient information, Caroline broadened the idea of column topics for the Review Matrix. She used the broad headings of the three-part series to develop three subtopics, consisting of research studies, interviews (further subdivided by parents, day care providers, regulators, experts, and other), and statistical findings. In constructing the Review Matrix, Caroline treated each type of information as a document, whether it was a research study, a set of notes on a standardized interview form, or a list of statistical findings. By using the Review Matrix in this way, she was better able to see what was missing and where she needed additional information. Throughout this process, Caroline also tracked the numbers of documents at each stage of the research process. She added the numbers to the PRISMA Flowchart.[1] Caroline then wrote a brief three-page memo synthesizing the information using the Review Matrix—one page for each of the three intended articles.

While she was in the process of preparing the Master Folder on day care injuries, Caroline also used the Matrix Indexing System to either download information from an electronic source, such as MEDLINE, or enter notes directly into a word processing document on her computer. In addition to the standard EndNote templates for a journal article, book, or report, Caroline also had the option of using a template for a newspaper article, a personal communication (which she used to record each of the interviews), and a generic format that she used to make a record of her statistical reports.

As they were going over the final materials in preparation for writing the three-part series, Caroline's reporter mentor was surprised by the effort Caroline had gone to in organizing the background information. "This is a lot of work!" her mentor commented. "Usually I just keep a few notes on a yellow legal pad from which I write the article."

"I know it seems like extra effort," Caroline replied, "but actually it's a lot easier to have it all in the same place in the Master Folder—where I can just grab the whole set when I need it. Storing everything in a Master Folder, together with a downloaded copy of each article in the Source Documents Subfolder, also helps me keep track of where things are for other writing assignments. I can't always remember where I put a downloaded copy of a study or the notes of an interview, but I can usually recall which assignment I was working on. Then all I have to do is go to the Master Folder on that assignment. It's called the Matrix Method."

Caroline's mentor commented, "Seems to me that the Matrix Method is useful in a lot of ways when it is necessary to summarize information. I think I'll try it myself."

"Oh, yes," Caroline said a bit smugly, "it's a very useful strategy. Even from the beginning, I knew the Matrix Method was more than just a simple spreadsheet that's called a Review Matrix."

Caroline raised her eyebrows a bit like Professor Dickerson did when he began a lecture, "The Matrix Method is a system for how to access, integrate, and use information from a variety of sources to prepare a written synthesis of the literature. I recommend it highly."

REFERENCES

1. Moher D, Liberati A, Tetzlaff J, Altman DG; The PRISMA Group. Preferred reporting items for systematic reviews and meta-analyses: the PRISMA Statement. *BMJ*. 2009;339:b2535. doi:http://dx.doi.org/10.1136/bmj.b2535.
2. Guyatt GH, Rennie D. Users' guides to the medical literature. *JAMA*. 1993;270:2096-2097.
3. Oxman AD, Sackett DL, Guyatt GH. Users' guides to the medical literature: I: how to get started. *JAMA*. 1993;270:2093-2095.
4. Guyatt GH, Sackett DL, Cook DJ; for the Evidence-Based Medicine Working Group. Users' guides to the medical literature: II: how to use an article about therapy or prevention: A: are the results of the study valid? *JAMA*. 1993;270:2598-2601.
5. Guyatt GH, Sackett DL, Cook DJ; for the Evidence-Based Medicine Working Group. Users' guides to the medical literature: II: how to use an article about therapy or prevention: B: what were the results and will they help me in caring for my patients? *JAMA*. 1994;271:59-63.
6. Jaeschke R, Guyatt G, Sackett DL; for the Evidence-Based Medicine Working Group. Users' guides to the medical literature: III: how to use an article about a diagnostic test: A: are the results of the study valid? *JAMA*. 1994;271:389-391.
7. Jaeschke R, Guyatt GH, Sackett DL; for the Evidence-Based Medicine Working Group. Users' guides to the medical literature: III: how to use an article about a diagnostic test: B: what are the results and will they help me in caring for my patients? *JAMA*. 1994;271:703-707.

8. Levine M, Walter S, Lee H, Haines T, Holbrook A, Moyer V; for the Evidence-Based Medicine Working Group. Users' guides to the medical literature: IV: how to use an article about harm. *JAMA*. 1994;271:1615-1619.

9. Laupacis A, Wells G, Richardson WS, Tugwell P; for the Evidence-Based Medicine Working Group. Users' guides to the medical literature: V: how to use an article about prognosis. *JAMA*. 1994;272:234-237.

10. Oxman AD, Cook DJ, Guyatt GH; for the Evidence-Based Medicine Working Group. Users' guides to the medical literature: VI: how to use an overview. *JAMA*. 1994; 272:1367-1371.

11. Richardson WS, Detsky AS; for the Evidence-Based Medicine Working Group. Users' guides to the medical literature: VII: how to use a clinical decision analysis: A: are the results of the study valid? *JAMA*. 1995;273:1292-1295.

12. Richardson WS, Detsky AS; for the Evidence-Based Medicine Working Group. Users' guides to the medical literature: VII: how to use a clinical decision analysis: B: what are the results and will they help me in caring for my patients? *JAMA*. 1995;273: 1610-1613.

13. Hayward RS, Wilson MC, Tunis SR, Bass EB, Guyatt G; for the Evidence-Based Medicine Working Group. Users' guides to the medical literature: VIII: how to use clinical practice guidelines: A: are the recommendations valid? *JAMA*. 1995;274:570-574.

14. Wilson MC, Hayward RS, Tunis SR, Bass EB, Guyatt G; for the Evidence-Based Medicine Working Group. Users' guides to the medical literature: VIII: how to use clinical practice guidelines: B: what are the recommendations and will they help you in caring for your patients? *JAMA*. 1995;274:1630-1632.

15. Guyatt GH, Sackett DL, Sinclair JC, Hayward R, Cook DJ, Cook RJ. Users' guides to the medical literature: IX: a method for grading health care recommendations. *JAMA*. 1995;274:1800-1804.

16. Naylor CD, Guyatt GH; for the Evidence-Based Medicine Working Group. Users' guides to the medical literature: X: how to use an article reporting variations in the outcomes of health services. *JAMA*. 1996;275:554-558.

17. Naylor CD, Guyatt GH; for the Evidence-Based Medicine Working Group. Users' guides to the medical literature: XI: how to use an article about a clinical utilization review. *JAMA*. 1996;275:1435-1439.

18. Guyatt GH, Naylor CD, Juniper E, Heyland DK, Jaeschke R, Cook DJ; for the Evidence-Based Medicine Working Group. Users' guides to the medical literature: XII: how to use articles about health-related quality of life. *JAMA*. 1997;277:1232-1237.

19. Drummond MG, Richardson WS, O'Brien BJ, Levine M, Heyland D; for the Evidence-Based Medicine Working Group. Users' guides to the medical literature: XIII: how to use an article on economic analysis of clinical practice: A: are the results of the study valid? *JAMA*. 1997;277:1552-1557.

20. O'Brien BJ, Heyland D, Richardson WS, Levine M, Drummond MF; for the Evidence-Based Medicine Working Group. Users' guides to the medical literature: XIII: how to use an article on economic analysis of clinical practice: B: what are the results and will they help me in caring for my patients? *JAMA*. 1997;277:1802-1806.

21. Dans AL, Dans LF, Guyatt GH, Richardson S; for the Evidence-Based Medicine Working Group. Users' guides to the medical literature: XIV: how to decide on the applicability of clinical trial results to your patient. *JAMA*. 1998;279:545-549.

22. Richardson WS, Wilson MC, Guyatt GH, Cook DJ, Nishikawa J; for the Evidence-Based Medicine Working Group. Users' guides to the medical literature:

XV: how to use an article about disease probability for differential diagnosis. *JAMA*. 1999;281:1214-1219.

23. Guyatt GH, Sinclair J, Cook DJ, Glasziou P; for the Evidence-Based Medicine Working Group and the Cochrane Applicability Methods Working Group. Users' guides to the medical literature: XVI: how to use a treatment recommendation. *JAMA*. 1999; 281:1836-1843.

24. Barratt A, Irwig L, Glasziou P, et al.; for the Evidence-Based Medicine Working Group. Users' guides to the medical literature: XVII: how to use guidelines and recommendations about screening. *JAMA*. 1999;281:2029-2034.

25. Randolph AG, Haynes RB, Wyatt JC, Cook DJ, Guyatt GH; for the Evidence-Based Medicine Working Group. Users' guides to the medical literature: XVIII: how to use an article evaluating the clinical impact of a computer-based clinical decision support system. *JAMA*. 1999;282:67-74.

26. Bucher HC, Guyatt GH, Cook DJ, Holbrook A, McAlister FA; for the Evidence-Based Medicine Working Group. Users' guides to the medical literature: XIX: applying clinical trial results: A: how to use an article measuring the effect of an intervention on surrogate end points. *JAMA*. 1999;282:771-778.

27. McAlister FA, Laupacis A, Wells GA, Sackett DL; for the Evidence-Based Medicine Working Group. Users' guides to the medical literature: XIX: applying clinical trial results: B: guidelines for determining whether a drug is exerting (more than) a class effect. *JAMA*. 1999;282:1371-1377.

28. Hunt DL, Jaeschke R, McKibbon KA; for the Evidence-Based Medicine Working Group. Users' guides to the medical literature: XXI: using electronic health information resources in evidence-based practice. *JAMA*. 2000;283:1875-1879.

29. McAlister FA, Straus SE, Guyatt GH, Haynes RB; for the Evidence-Based Medicine Working Group. Users' guides to the medical literature: XX: integrating research evidence with the care of the individual patient. *JAMA*. 2000;283:2829-2836.

30. McGinn TG, Guyatt GH, Wyer PC, Naylor CD, Stiell IG, Richardson WS; for the Evidence-Based Medicine Working Group. Users' guides to the medical literature: XXII: how to use articles about clinical decision rules. *JAMA*. 2000;284:79-84.

31. Giacomini MK, Cook DJ; for the Evidence-Based Medicine Working Group. Users' guides to the medical literature: XXIII: qualitative research in health care: B: what are the results and how do they help me care for my patients? *JAMA*. 2000;284:478-482.

32. Richardson WS, Wilson MC, Williams JW Jr, Moyer VA, Naylor CD; for the Evidence-Based Medicine Working Group. Users' guides to the medical literature: XXIV: how to use an article on the clinical manifestations of disease. *JAMA*. 2000; 284:869-875.

33. Guyatt GH, Haynes RB, Jaeschke RZ, et al. Users' guides to the medical literature: XXV: evidence-based medicine: principles for applying the users' guides to patient care. *JAMA*. 2000;284:1290-1296.

34. Strauman-Raymond K, Lie L, Kempf-Berkseth J. Creating a safe environment for children in day care. *J School Health*. 1993;63:254-257.

35. Bernardo LM. Parent-reported injury-associated behaviors and life events among injured, ill, and well preschool children. *J Pediatr Nursing*. 1996;11:100-110.

36. Williams AF, Wells JAK, Ferguson SA. Development and evaluation of programs to increase proper child restraint use. *J Safety Res*. 1997;28:197-202.

Useful Resources for Literature Reviews

PURPOSE

This appendix consists of lists of resources that may be useful in searching for information as you review the literature. Websites, as well as print sources, are provided. The website addresses were accurate at the time this edition was published, but they can change; the author and publisher assume no responsibility for their continued accuracy. If the address is not accurate when you use it, try using the key words of the organization in a general search for the correct address.

REFERENCES AND WEBSITES FOR HEALTH SCIENCES PROFESSIONALS

National Academies of Sciences, Engineering, and Medicine:
http://www.nationalacademies.org/hmd/About-HMD.aspx

In March 2016, the name of the Institute of Medicine was changed to the Health and Medicine Division of the National Academies of Science, Engineering, and Medicine. Go to this online source to see IOM reports as well as HMD reports.

Evidence-Based Clinical Practice Guidelines:
http://www.guideline.gov/index.aspx

The National Guideline Clearinghouse (NGC) is a public resource that includes the Evidence-Based Clinical Practice Guidelines. The NGC includes much more in terms of resources, a comparison of guidelines, and other information. This is described in Chapter 1 of this book.

Print Sources

American Medical Association. *Clinical Practice Guidelines Directory: 1999–2000 Ed.* Chicago, IL: American Medical Association; 2000.

Green E, Katz J, eds. *Clinical Practice Guidelines for the Adult Patient.* St. Louis, MO: Mosby; 1994.

Lechtenberg R, Schutta HS, eds. *Neurology Practice Guidelines.* New York, NY: M. Dekker; 1998.

National Comprehensive Cancer Network. Oncology practice guidelines. *Oncology.* 1996;10(suppl 11):3-317.

U.S. Preventive Services Task Force. *Guide to Clinical Preventive Services: Recommendations of the U.S. Preventive Services Task Force.* 3rd ed. Washington, DC: Agency for Healthcare Research and Quality; 2005. http://www.ahrq.gov/clinic/uspstfix.htm

Clinical Practice Guidelines

Centers for Disease Control and Prevention. *Morbidity and Mortality Weekly Report (MMWR).* http://www.cdc.gov/mmwr

U.S. Preventive Services Task Force. *Guide to Clinical Preventive Services: Recommendations of the U.S. Preventive Services Task Force.* 3rd ed. Washington, DC: Agency for Healthcare Research and Quality; 2005. http://www.ahrq.gov/clinic/uspstfix.htm

Additional References About Clinical Guidelines

Cook DJ, Greengold NL, Ellrodt AG, Weingarten SR. The relations between systematic reviews and practice guidelines. *Ann Intern Med.* 1997;127:210-216.

Field MJ, Lohr KN, eds. *Guidelines for Clinical Practice: From Development to Use.* Institute of Medicine, Washington, DC: National Academy Press; 1992. This 1992 edition of the book is available online (http://www.nap.edu/read/1863/chapter/1).

Lohr KN. Guidelines for clinical practice: what they are and why they count. *J Law Med Ethics.* 1995;23:49-56.

Saver, BG. Whose guideline is it, anyway [editorial]? *Arch Fam Med.* 1996;5:532-534.

Evidence-Based Medicine: List of Users' Guides by Year of Publication

1993 Users' Guides

Guyatt GH, Rennie D. Users' guides to the medical literature [editorial]. *JAMA.* 1993;270:2096-2097.

Guyatt GH, Sackett DL, Cook DJ, for the Evidence-Based Medicine Working Group. Users' guides to the medical literature: II: how to use an article about therapy or prevention: A: are the results of the study valid? *JAMA.* 1993;270:2598-2601.

Oxman AD, Sackett DL, Guyatt GH. Users' guides to the medical literature: I: how to get started. *JAMA.* 1993;270:2093-2095.

1994 Users' Guides

Guyatt GH, Sackett DL, Cook DJ, for the Evidence-Based Medicine Working Group. Users' guides to the medical literature: II: how to use an article about therapy or prevention: B: what were the results and will they help me in caring for my patients? *JAMA*. 1994;271:59-63.

Jaeschke R, Guyatt G, Sackett DL, for the Evidence-Based Medicine Working Group. Users' guides to the medical literature: III: how to use an article about a diagnostic test: A: are the results of the study valid? *JAMA*. 1994;271:389-391.

Jaeschke R, Guyatt GH, Sackett DL, for the Evidence-Based Medicine Working Group. Users' guides to the medical literature: III: how to use an article about a diagnostic test: B: what are the results and will they help me in caring for my patients? *JAMA*. 1994;271:703-707.

Laupacis A, Wells G, Richardson WS, Tugwell P, for the Evidence-Based Medicine Working Group. Users' guides to the medical literature: V: how to use an article about prognosis. *JAMA*. 1994;272:234-237.

Levine M, Walter S, Lee H, et al., for the Evidence-Based Medicine Working Group. Users' guides to the medical literature: IV: how to use an article about harm. *JAMA*. 1994;271:1615-1619.

Oxman AD, Cook DJ, Guyatt GH, for the Evidence-Based Medicine Working Group. Users' guides to the medical literature: VI: how to use an overview. *JAMA*. 1994;272:1367-1371.

1995 Users' Guides

Guyatt GH, Sackett DL, Sinclair JC, et al., for the Evidence-Based Medicine Working Group. Users' guides to the medical literature: IX: a method for grading health care recommendations. *JAMA*. 1995;274:1800-1804.

Hayward RS, Wilson MC, Tunis SR, Bass EB, Guyatt G, for the Evidence-Based Medicine Working Group. Users' guides to the medical literature: VIII: how to use clinical practice guidelines: A: are the recommendations valid? *JAMA*. 1995;274:570-574.

Richardson WS, Detsky AS, for the Evidence-Based Medicine Working Group. Users' guides to the medical literature: VII: how to use a clinical decision analysis: A: are the results of the study valid? *JAMA*. 1995;273:1292-1295.

Richardson WS, Detsky AS, for the Evidence-Based Medicine Working Group. Users' guides to the medical literature: VII: how to use a clinical decision analysis: B: what are the results and will they help me in caring for my patients? *JAMA*. 1995;273:1610-1613.

Wilson MC, Hayward RS, Tunis SR, Bass EB, Guyatt G, for the Evidence-Based Medicine Working Group. Users' guides to the medical literature: VIII: how to use clinical practice guidelines: B: what are the recommendations and will they help you in caring for your patients? *JAMA*. 1995;274:1630-1632.

1996 Users' Guides

Naylor CD, Guyatt GH, for the Evidence-Based Medicine Working Group. Users' guides to the medical literature: X: how to use an article reporting variations in the outcomes of health services. *JAMA*. 1996;275:554-558.

Naylor CD, Guyatt GH, for the Evidence-Based Medicine Working Group. Users' guides to the medical literature: XI: how to use an article about a clinical utilization review. *JAMA*. 1996;275:1435-1439.

1997 Users' Guides

Drummond MG, Richardson WS, O'Brien BJ, Levine M, Heyland D, for the Evidence-Based Medicine Working Group. Users' guides to the medical literature: XIII: how to use an article on economic analysis of clinical practice: A: are the results of the study valid? *JAMA.* 1997;277:1552-1557.

Guyatt GH, Naylor CD, Juniper E, for the Evidence-Based Medicine Working Group. Users' guides to the medical literature: XII: how to use articles about health-related quality of life. *JAMA.* 1997;277:1232-1237.

O'Brien BJ, Heyland D, Richardson WS, Levine M, Drummond MF, for the Evidence-Based Medicine Working Group. Users' guides to the medical literature: XIII: how to use an article on economic analysis of clinical practice: B: what are the results and will they help me in caring for my patients? *JAMA.* 1997;277:1802-1806.

1998 Users' Guide

Dans AL, Dans LF, Guyatt GH, Richardson S, for the Evidence-Based Medicine Working Group. Users' guides to the medical literature: XIV: how to decide on the applicability of clinical trial results to your patient. *JAMA.* 1998;279:545-549.

1999 Users' Guides

Barratt A, Irwig L, Glasziou P, et al., for the Evidence-Based Medicine Working Group. Users' guides to the medical literature: XVII: how to use guidelines and recommendations about screening. *JAMA.* 1999;281:2029-2034.

Bucher HC, Guyatt GH, Cook DJ, Holbrook A, McAlister FA, for the Evidence-Based Medicine Working Group. Users' guides to the medical literature: XIX: applying clinical trial results: A: how to use an article measuring the effect of an intervention on surrogate end points. *JAMA.* 1999;282:771-778.

Guyatt GH, Sinclair J, Cook DJ, Glasziou P, for the Evidence-Based Medicine Working Group and the Cochrane Applicability Methods Working Group. Users' guides to the medical literature: XVI: how to use a treatment recommendation. *JAMA.* 1999;281:1836-1843.

McAlister FA, Laupacis A, Wells GA, Sackett DL, for the Evidence-Based Medicine Working Group. Users' guides to the medical literature: XIX: applying clinical trial results: B: guidelines for determining whether a drug is exerting (more than) a class effect. *JAMA.* 1999;282:1371-1377.

Randolph AG, Haynes RB, Wyatt JC, Cook DJ, Guyatt GH, for the Evidence-Based Medicine Working Group. Users' guides to the medical literature: XVIII: how to use an article evaluating the clinical impact of a computer-based clinical decision support system. *JAMA.* 1999;282:67-74.

Richardson WS, Wilson MC, Guyatt GH, Cook DJ, Nishikawa J, for the Evidence-Based Medicine Working Group. Users' guides to the medical literature: XV: how to use an article about disease probability for differential diagnosis. *JAMA.* 1999;281:1214-1219.

2000 Users' Guides

Giacomini MK, Cook DJ, for the Evidence-Based Medicine Working Group. Users' guides to the medical literature: XXIII: qualitative research in health care: A: are the results of the study valid? *JAMA.* 2000;284:357-362.

Guyatt GH, Haynes RB, Jaeschke RZ, Cook DJ, Green L, Naylor CD, Wilson MC, Richardson WS, for the Evidence-Based Medicine Working Group. Users' guides to the medical literature: XXV: evidence-based medicine: principles for applying the users' guides to patient care. *JAMA.* 2000;284:1290-1296.

Hunt DL, Jaeschke R, McKibbon KA, for the Evidence-Based Medicine Working Group. Users' guides to the medical literature: XXI: using electronic health information resources in evidence-based practice. *JAMA.* 2000;283:1875-1879.

McAlister FA, Straus SE, Guyatt GH, Haynes RB, for the Evidence-Based Medicine Working Group. Users' guides to the medical literature: XX: integrating research evidence with the care of the individual patient. *JAMA.* 2000;283:2829-2836.

McGinn TG, Guyatt GH, Wyer PC, Naylor CD, Stiell IG, Richardson WS, for the Evidence-Based Medicine Working Group. Users' guides to the medical literature: XXII: how to use articles about clinical decision rules. *JAMA.* 2000;284:79-84.

Richardson WS, Wilson MC, Williams JW Jr, Moyer VA, Naylor CD, for the Evidence-Based Medicine Working Group. Users' guides to the medical literature: XXIV: how to use an article on the clinical manifestations of disease. *JAMA.* 2000;284: 869-875.

Users' Guides Published after 2000

For an updated list of users' guides published after 2000, consult the following book:
Guyatt G, Rennie D, Meade MO, Cook DJ. *Users' Guides to the Medical Literature: A Manual for Evidence-Based Clinical Practice.* 2nd ed. New York, NY: McGraw-Hill Companies/American Medical Association; 2008.

Cochrane Reviews

A list of reviews is available at the Cochrane Collaboration website: http://www.cochrane.org

Annual Reviews by Category

Reviews of scientific information are published annually by Annual Reviews, which is a nonprofit scientific publisher. Current information about reviews can be found at the following website: http://www.annualreviews.org. Currently, there are 41 annual reviews in three categories, biomedical/life sciences, physical sciences, and social sciences. For an up-to-date list of all Annual Reviews publications, go to the following website: http://www.annualreviews.org. To see the names of the journals, pull down the tab, Journals, at the top of the page.

Useful Print Resources

Boorkman JA, Huber JT, Roper FW. *Introduction to Reference Sources in the Health Sciences.* 4th ed. New York, NY: Neal-Schuman Publishers; 2004.

Bopp RE, Smith LC. *Reference and Information Services: An Introduction.* 2nd ed. Englewood, CO: Libraries Unlimited; 1995.

Kuhlthau CC. *Seeking Meaning: A Process Approach to Library and Information Services.* Norwood, NJ: Ablex Publishing; 1993.

Kuhlthau CC. *Teaching the Library Research Process.* 2nd ed. Metuchen, NJ: The Scarecrow Press; 1994.

Lamm K. *10,000 Ideas for Term Papers, Projects, Reports & Speeches.* New York, NY: Macmillan; 1995.

Websites of Scientific Organizations, Directories, Printed Journals, and Online Journals

American Anthropological Association (http://www.americananthro.org). Homepage of the American Anthropological Association.

American Association for the Advancement of Science (http://www.aaas.org). Homepage of the American Association for the Advancement of Science (AAAS). Includes links and information to many science fields.

American Chemical Society (http://www.chemistry.org). Homepage of the American Chemical Society, with a membership of more than 157,000 chemists and chemical engineers.

American Institute of Biological Sciences (http://www.aibs.org). Homepage of the American Institute of Biological Sciences, with links to *BioScience Magazine.*

American Journal of Clinical Nutrition (http://ajcn.nutrition.org). Homepage of the *American Journal of Clinical Nutrition,* which is a peer-reviewed journal that publishes basic and clinical studies relevant to human nutrition.

American Society for Biochemistry and Molecular Biology (http://www.asbmb.org). Homepage of the American Society for Biochemistry and Molecular Biology.

American Society of Human Genetics (http://www.ashg.org). Homepage of the American Society of Human Genetics.

American Sociological Association (http://www.asanet.org). Homepage of the American Sociological Association.

Association for Psychological Science (http://www.psychologicalscience.org). Homepage for the Psychological Science journals.

BankIt: GenBank Submissions by WWW (http://www.ncbi.nlm.nih.gov/genbank /update). Site for submitting genetic sequences and information on protein coding regions, mRNA features, and structural RNA features to the GenBank library. The website is currently under revision.

CABI (http://www.cabi.org). Emphasis on agriculture, forestry, human health, and the management of natural resources, with particular attention to the needs of developing countries.

Center for Advancing Health (CFAH) (http://www.cfah.org). The mission statement is as follows: "CFAH conducts research, communicates findings and advocates for policies that support everyone's ability to benefit from advances in health science."

Federation of American Societies for Experimental Biology (http://www.faseb.org). Homepage of the Federation of American Societies for Experimental Biology.

International Sociological Association (http://www.isa-sociology.org). Homepage of the International Sociological Association.

Journal of Biological Chemistry (http://www.jbc.org). Online version of the *Journal of Biological Chemistry.*

Journal of Cell Biology (http://jcb.rupress.org). Online version of the *Journal of Cell Biology.*

Journal of Clinical Investigation (http://www.jci.org). Online version of the *Journal of Clinical Investigation.*

Journal of Experimental Medicine (http://jem.rupress.org). Online version of the *Journal of Experimental Medicine.*

Journal of Nutrition (http://nutrition.org). Published by the American Society for Nutrition. Online version of the *Journal of Nutrition,* which publishes papers based on original research in humans and other animal species.

Journal Watch (http://www.jwatch.org). Journal Watch began in 1987 in both an online and newsletter format. It reviews the general medical literature for busy clinicians.

National Center for Biotechnology Information (http://www.ncbi.nlm.nih.gov). A searchable molecular biology subset of MEDLINE with more than 1.5 million citations.

Science (http://www.sciencemag.org). Homepage of *Science Magazine Online* with full text of print edition and science news section.

ScienceCareers.org (http://www.sciencemag.org/careers). A site for helping new scientists find jobs and keep up with new developments in their careers.

Society for Neuroscience (http://www.sfn.org). Focuses on understanding the brain and nervous system.

SocioSite (http://www.sociosite.net). Site for sociologists with a European and world-wide horizon. This Social Science Information System is located at the University of Amsterdam.

Thomson Reuters Scholarly & Scientific Research (http://thomsonreuters.com/en /products-services/scholarly-scientific-research.html). Publisher of Current Contents Connect (http://thomsonreuters.com/en/products-services/scholarly-scientific-research/ scholarly-search-and-discovery/current-contents-connect.html), WebofScience, which includes Science Citation Index (http://ipscience.thomsonreuters.com/product/web -of-science/?utm_source=Adwords&utm_medium=paid&utm_campaign=WoS), ScienceWatch (http://sciencewatch.com), and EndNote (http://endnote.com).

Structure
of Computer
Folders for the
Matrix Method

This appendix provides you with step-by-step instructions for creating a structure of folders for the Matrix Method on your computer. These instructions assume you want to set up an arrangement of folders and blank documents before you begin your review of the literature. At the end of this appendix, there are answers to frequently asked questions about some of these suggestions and a complete example of the infrastructure of folders and files.

FOLDER STRUCTURE

Master Folder

Create a Master Folder for each literature review you conduct. Include a one- or two-word descriptor as the topic for each Master Folder. For example, if you are planning to conduct two separate literature reviews, one on the public health effects of flooding and the other on prevention of malaria, then you would have two Master Folders:

Master Folder—Flooding

Master Folder—Malaria

Four Main Folders in the Master Folder

In each Master Folder, include four folders corresponding to the four major parts of the Matrix Method. Include the topic label after each. Here are two examples:

Master Folder—Flooding
    Paper Trail Folder—Flooding
    Documents Folder—Flooding
    Review Matrix Folder—Flooding
    Synthesis Folder—Flooding

Master Folder—Malaria
    Paper Trail Folder—Malaria
    Documents Folder—Malaria
    Review Matrix Folder—Malaria
    Synthesis Folder—Malaria

Within each of the four main folders in the Master Folder, you will place additional documents or subfolders as you progress through the Matrix Method. Here are some suggestions for your labeling of the folders in the initial setup.

Paper Trail Folder

In the Paper Trail Folder, create five word processing documents. These will be blank at first, but you will use them to store notes as you progress through your review of the literature. Because you are creating them all at once, it will be easy to add the topic name when saving each document.

Paper Trail Folder—topic
    Key Words Subfolder—topic
    Resources Subfolder—topic
    Bibliographic Databases Subfolder—topic
    Internet Documents Subfolder—topic
    Miscellaneous Notes Subfolder—topic

Documents Folder

In the Documents Folder, you will create two main subfolders: the Source Documents Subfolder and the PRISMA Flowchart Subfolder. The Source Documents is the place where you will store all of the pdfs of journal articles and other source materials you download in your review of the literature. If the review of the literature contains source documents that span several decades, I find it easiest to create additional subfolders in the Source Documents Subfolder by decade of publication. Thus, if the literature review extends from 1980 to the present,

I might create four subfolders for papers published between 1980 and 1989, between 1990 and 1999, from 2000 to 2009, and from 2010 to the present. Of course I label each folder as follows:

Source Documents Subfolder—topic
    Source Documents Subfolder—topic, 1980–89
    Source Documents Subfolder—topic, 1990–99
    Source Documents Subfolder—topic, 2000–09
    Source Documents Subfolder—topic, 2010–present

Other ways of storing these documents could be used. For example, if you were organizing the papers in a literature review of the public health effects of flooding, you might organize by age of victim (infants, children, adults, elderly) or by global area in which the flooding occurred (North America, Central America, South America, Western Europe, other areas). Your goal in creating these subfolders is to have a well-understood location for storing the large number of studies you are likely to download in your review of the literature.

Review Matrix Folder

In conducting a literature review, you will create a Review Matrix. Initially, when this was a paper-and-pencil system, there was only one matrix, which couldn't be easily reorganized. Now your Review Matrix is stored on the computer and can be sorted however you wish, especially if it is based on a spreadsheet program such as Microsoft Excel or the table option in Microsoft Word. Your Review Matrix Subfolder and Synthesis Subfolder are the two most important products of your Review of the Literature based on the Matrix Method. For that reason, you will use the same format for each of these two subfolders as shown in this section on the Review Matrix and the following section on Synthesis.

Review Matrix Folder—topic
    Review Matrix CURRENT Subfolder—topic—9-24-16
        Initially, you will place the first draft of the Review Matrix (9-20-16-original) in the Review Matrix CURRENT Subfolder. The next time you revise that draft and change to the current date, you will move the first draft to the Review Matrix PREVIOUS Subfolder, and work on the most current draft, e.g., 9-24-16. There should be only one draft of the Review Matrix in the Review Matrix CURRENT Subfolder at any time.
    Review Matrix PREVIOUS Subfolder—topic—9-20-16-original
        Remember to keep a copy of all your previous drafts stored in this PREVIOUS subfolder. Thus this subfolder will have a large number of previous drafts.
    Review Matrix FINAL Subfolder—topic—9-28-16 final

When you have the final draft of the Review Matrix, store it in this subfolder. The Review Matrix FINAL Subfolder should have only one draft—the final product.

Synthesis Folder

The Synthesis Folder is where you will keep a copy of all versions of your synthesis. At the end of each working session or day, save your current draft of the synthesis, date stamp, and store in the Synthesis CURRENT Subfolder. (See chapter 6.) Here is an example of some drafts of the synthesis documents you would store in this folder:

Synthesis Folder—topic

Synthesis CURRENT Subfolder—topic—7-24-16

Initially, you will place the first draft of the synthesis (7-20-16-original) in the Synthesis CURRENT Subfolder. The next time you revise that draft and change to the current date, you will move the first draft to the Synthesis PREVIOUS Subfolder, and work on the most current draft, e.g., 7-24-16. There should be only one draft of the synthesis in the Synthesis CURRENT Subfolder at any time.

Synthesis PREVIOUS Subfolder—topic—7-20-16 original

Remember to keep a copy of all your previous drafts stored in this PREVIOUS subfolder. Thus this subfolder will have a large number of previous drafts.

Synthesis FINAL Subfolder—topic—7-28-16 final

When you have written the final draft of the synthesis, store it in this subfolder. The Synthesis FINAL Subfolder should have only one draft—the final product.

FREQUENTLY ASKED QUESTIONS

1. **Why repeat the topic on the folders or files?**
   Documents can get lost or mistakenly assigned to other folders, sometimes with an accidental flick of the wrist. By routinely adding a topic tag to your folders or files, you can always use the Find command to locate errant files.

2. **Why should I keep different drafts of the synthesis? Why not continually modify the original version and keep that version?**
   The first draft of the synthesis can often be a brain dump or a stream of consciousness narrative of the review. Generally I use a no-holds-barred approach in writing this draft—with no page limits and usually very little editing. Sometimes there are creative insights in the original draft that I may not use when I edit the second or later drafts.

   In general, store all of your previous drafts in the Synthesis PREVIOUS Subfolder (see chapter 6 in this book). Don't edit over them because you may edit out some of the details you wish you had later. By saving the original and each of the rewrites, you preserve that information.

3. **How can I easily identify these Master Folders?**
Most word processing systems have a feature that allows the user to color code a file or document. I find it useful to assign the same color to all the Master Folders, and this allows me to easily find them on my desktop.

4. **Why would I want to assemble the Review Matrix Folders from different literature reviews?**
If you have two or more Master Folders, you can compare the content of the same folders, syntheses, or documents, across these different literature reviews. For example, on your desktop you might have completed four literature reviews on different but related topics. You might decide to compare the Review Matrices across those topics. Because you have used the same title for the first three words for those documents, you could use the Find command to locate "Review Matrix original." You would also be able to restore these files to their original folders by noting the topic name.

Another possibility might be to compare different documents, syntheses, or folders across collaborators. For example, a team of five people working on a practice guideline in hand-washing techniques might want to compare the methods sort of their different review matrices prior to writing a synthesis together. By putting a copy of the complete Master Folder by each team member on the same desktop (and tagging each file or folder with the person's identification), their Review Matrix and methods sort spreadsheets could be pulled together and compared. They could then be restored to their original folders when the task is done.

5. **Why should I set up this elaborate structure of folders and subfolders when all I have to do is write up the results of a review of the literature?**
A review of the literature can be a multiday, multiweek process that requires time, thought, and organization. You need a plan for where to put your tools and your products as you progress toward completion of a synthesis. The reason to set up a structure of folders and files before you start your review is that otherwise things get lost or merged or not saved at all as you navigate this complex task.

Creating a structure of folders and files is like building a set of shelves in a kitchen. When you cook a large meal, you need to know where the equipment is or can be stored, where the food is located, and where to put different dishes, such as the salad in the refrigerator and the hot dish in the oven before the meal is served. That infrastructure of shelves, appliances, and an understanding of the layout of the kitchen itself contribute to your getting the meal on the table. Enjoy!

EXAMPLE OF FILE STRUCTURE
FOR THE MATRIX METHOD

Master Folder—Flooding
   Paper Trail Folder—Flooding
      Key Words Subfolder—Flooding
      Resources Subfolder—Flooding
      Bibliographic Databases Subfolder—Flooding
      Internet Documents Subfolder—Flooding
      Miscellaneous Notes Subfolder—Flooding

Documents Folder—Flooding
   Source Documents Subfolder—Flooding
      (Organize all source documents chronologically by year of publication in the Source Documents Subfolder.)
   PRISMA Flowchart Subfolder

Review Matrix Folder—Flooding
   Review Matrix CURRENT Subfolder—Flooding
   Review Matrix PREVIOUS Subfolder—Flooding
   Review Matrix FINAL Subfolder—Flooding

Synthesis Folder—Flooding
   Synthesis CURRENT Subfolder—Flooding
   Synthesis PREVIOUS Subfolder—Flooding
   Synthesis FINAL Subfolder—Flooding

In general, the structure you are setting up differs depending on the folder or subfolder you are using. For example, in the Paper Trail Folder and in the Synthesis Folder, you mainly will use word processing documents. In the Review Matrix Folder you will use either spreadsheet documents or word processing documents using the table option of Word. And in the Source Documents Subfolder (located in the Documents Folder), you will use Word Documents or Excel files.

Although you can create a skeleton structure for the contents of the Paper Trail Folder and the Documents Folder before you start the actual literature review, bear in mind that what you include in the Review Matrix Folder and the Synthesis Folder will be created as your work progresses. It is good to set up this infrastructure in advance, but it is also helpful to know what else you need to do in the process of going through the Matrix Method.

Data Visualization: A Digital Exploration

To access Appendix C, visit http://www.jblearning.com and redeem the access code at the front of your book.

Index

Exhibits and figures are indicated by an italic *f* following the page number.